TRANSFORMING
HEALTH CARE
LEADERSHIP

TRANSFORMING HEALTH CARE LEADERSHIP

A Systems Guide to Improve Patient Care, Decrease Costs, and Improve Population Health

MICHAEL MACCOBY

CLIFFORD L. NORMAN

C. JANE NORMAN

RICHARD MARGOLIES

JB JOSSEY-BASS™
A Wiley Brand

Published by Jossey-Bass
A Wiley Brand
One Montgomery Street, Suite 1200, San Francisco, CA 94104–4594 www.josseybass.com

Jossey-Bass books and products are available through most bookstores. To contact Jossey-Bass directly call our Customer Care Department within the U.S. at 800-956-7739, outside the U.S. at 317-572-3986, or fax 317-572-4002.

Wiley publishes in a variety of print and electronic formats and by print—on—demand. Some material included with standard print versions of this book may not be included in e-books or in print-on-demand. If this book refers to media such as a CD or DVD that is not included in the version you purchased, you may download this material at http://booksupport.wiley.com. For more information about Wiley products, visit www.wiley.com.

Library of Congress Cataloging-in-Publication Data

Transforming health care leadership : a systems guide to improve patient care, decrease costs, and improve population health / Michael Maccoby ... [et al.]. – 1st ed.
    p. ; cm.

    Includes bibliographical references and index.
        ISBN 978-1-118-50563-2 (hardback); ISBN 978-1-118-60399-4 (ebk.);
ISBN 978-1-118-60367-3 (ebk.); ISBN 978-1-118-60366-6 (ebk.)
    I. Maccoby, Michael
    [DNLM: 1.   Delivery of Health Care–organization & administration–United States.
   2.   Leadership–United States. 3.   Organizational Innovation–United States.   W 84 AA1]

    RA971.3
    362.1068–dc23   2013011323

Printed in the United States of America
FIRST EDITION
HB Printing   10 9 8 7 6 5 4 3 2 1

Contents

Part 3:
Learning from Other Leaders and Creating a Path Forward   191

List of Figures

List of Tables

List of Exhibits

Why and How We Wrote This Book

We wrote this book because our experience convinces us that with the right kind of leadership, health care organizations can improve patient care, decrease per capita cost, and improve community health; however, we also see that current models of leadership and conceptual tools for change are inadequate. The purpose of this book is to provide a practical guide for the kind of leadership needed. It combines concepts and tools, theory and proven practice.

Changes in products, processes, and organizational structure take place all the time as organizations grow or adapt to changing markets, technologies, government regulations, or restructure after mergers and acquisitions. But fundamentally transforming an organization is extremely difficult. However, there are three reasons why leaders take on the challenge:

To avoid imminent extinction: The organization is threatened with imminent extinction; it may be too late for survival in the present form. Options usually include bankruptcy, a leveraged buyout, and severe cost reduction strategies such as downsizing or simply choosing to do nothing and disappear. If the organization does survive, it will have to change.

To avoid threats that could seriously damage or destroy the organization: Leaders have the foresight to see that future threats will damage or destroy the organization, and they take the necessary action today to position the organization for adaptation to a better future.

To improve effectiveness: Visionary leaders can imagine how the organization can become more effective. An idealized design of the future is developed and becomes a shared vision for the organization.

This book presents leaders with the concepts and tools to use foresight, to create an idealized vision for the future, and to implement it.

The *Oxford English Dictionary* defines *transformation* as changing the form or altering the character of something. Note that this book is not titled transforming *leaders*, but rather transforming *leadership*. Although we describe the knowledge and understanding that leaders of health care need to develop, we set this development in the context of transforming an organization, a social system. Leadership implies a relationship between leaders and collaborators. An effective health care organization will have different types of leaders working interactively throughout the organization, mobilizing collaborators to continuously improve the system. This book not only describes the types of leaders and what they need to know and do, but it also explains why and how collaborators can become engaged in the transformation.

The transformation of leadership in this sense requires continuous improvement of processes as well as individuals. It requires leadership with constancy of purpose, not only at the strategic level, but also throughout a health care organization. The knowledge and tools presented in this book will challenge concepts and beliefs held by many managers. We list some of these beliefs or management myths in the Introduction. The improvements that can be achieved by using the concepts and tools described in this book require a great deal of time and work, but the potential returns are great in terms of patient well-being, productivity, and benefits to communities.

The authors of this book have a combined total of over fifty years of studying health care organizations and consulting to those attempting change. This guide is based on what we have observed from the most effective health care organizations and what we have helped construct in those organizations that have hired us.

We have come together from different paths. In 1988, Henry Simmons organized the National Commission on Health Care, and asked

Michael Maccoby to facilitate its meetings. The commission members included distinguished leaders from medicine, business, politics, universities, religious organizations, and unions. They heard testimony from economists and practitioners on the problems of rising costs, quality of care, and lack of insurance for over 15 percent of the U.S. population. In 1990, the Commission evolved into the National Coalition on Health Care (NCHC) and grew into nearly a hundred organizations, including provider groups, businesses, unions, pension funds, religious organizations, health care organizations, and insurers. Maccoby facilitated a number of meetings of the Coalition in 2003 that resulted in a consensus on the elements of a policy that would effectively address the problems of health care in America. In 2004, the Coalition published a report, *Building a Better Health Care System: Specifications for Reform*, that presented five principles or goals for a reformed health care system:

Health Care Coverage for All

Cost Management

Improvement of Health Care Quality and Safety

Equitable Financing

Simplified Administration

The Affordable Care Act (ACA) has moved toward these goals, but it has not taken the country the full distance. The way costs and pricing are determined raise issues for our society. NCHC continues to study and propose policies to improve care, decrease costs, and improve population health. Maccoby serves on the board of its Action Fund.

In the fall of 2012, under the leadership of John Rother, the Coalition presented a seven-point strategy designed to save money, improve care, and achieve better health outcomes:[1]

1. Change provider incentives to reward value, not volume
2. Encourage patient and consumer engagement
3. Use market competition to increase value
4. Ensure that the highest-cost patients receive high-value, coordinated care
5. Bolster the primary care workforce
6. Reduce errors, fraud, and administrative overhead
7. Invest in prevention and population health.

Maccoby came to these issues with experience as a practicing psychoanalyst and consultant to business and health care leaders who were working to improve productivity and the quality of working life. From this experience, he was convinced that no government policy could, by itself, cause health care organizations to improve quality and at the same time cut costs. To do so would require good leadership and improved processes. Furthermore, he saw a danger of health care organizations becoming static bureaucracies at a time when the most advanced knowledge companies were becoming dynamic learning organizations. The difference was one of mechanically delivering a standardized product versus coproducing, with customers, productive solutions that increased value for the customers. It was the difference between delivering care to passive patients versus coproducing health with active patients who shared responsibility for managing their own care and taking steps toward healthy living.

Two former classmates from Harvard College, Roger Bulger and Paul Griner, had become noted physicians and leaders of health care organizations. They encouraged Maccoby to study some of the best health care organizations in the United States and report on the kind of leadership required to continually improve productivity and the quality of care. They helped him to get a research grant from the Robert Wood Johnson Foundation and together with Simmons helped him gain entry into health care organizations they considered to be among the best in the United States. Results of the study are described in Chapter 2.

On the basis of this work, Maccoby was hired by leaders of four large health care organizations to aid them in attempts to transform their organizations. Richard Margolies, his principal research associate in the Robert Wood Johnson study, also assisted Maccoby when he was invited to help two health care organizations, described in Chapter 2, attempt to merge.

Cliff and Jane Norman assist their clients in developing, testing, and implementing process and management improvements. Their work typically involves helping clients understand their organizations as social systems to ensure that changes are aligned with strategy and executed effectively and efficiently. Cliff's first foray into health care in the late 1990s was helping Dayton Memorial Hospital view the work of the hospital as a system. In 2001, Cliff and Jane were asked to support the Robert Wood Johnson sponsored project on Pursuing Perfection in Jönköping, Sweden (see case in Chapter 10). They organized workshops on quality improvement and systems thinking and worked on specific improvement projects. Since then, they have worked with health care organizations in Canada, England, Scotland, Singapore, and many different parts of the United States.

Currently, the Normans are on the strategic advisory team of the Texas Team Advancing Health Through Nursing, an action coalition sponsored by the Robert Wood Johnson Foundation, AARP, and the Center to Champion Nursing in America under a campaign called the Future of Nursing: Campaign for Action. In addition, they support the work of Alexia Green at Texas Tech University Health Science Center, Lubbock, Texas, Doctorate of Nursing Practice Program. Jane recently held the position of COO for Our Community Health Information Network (OCHIN) where she has employed the ideas presented in this book as a practicing executive leader (see OCHIN case in Chapter 10).

In 2009, the Normans attended a workshop on leadership led by Maccoby and then invited him to present his ideas to the Southwest Quality Network of their clients who followed the improvement practices and theories advanced by W. Edwards Deming, Russell Ackoff, and others. Maccoby had been both a student and colleague of Deming and Ackoff and in 1990 had been invited by Deming to expand on his understanding of psychology and leadership. The Normans considered that Maccoby's concepts of strategic intelligence and psychology filled a gap in Deming's profound knowledge and could be combined with Deming's concepts of systems, understanding variation, theory of developing knowledge, and his methods of building a system of improvement and innovation. They suggested collaborating on this book, which is the result of integrating these concepts and their combined experience.

During the initial stages of learning and collaborating together, the Normans introduced Maccoby to the methods for leaders called "Quality as a Business Strategy," which had its foundation in Deming's idea of the organization viewed as a system. These methods were developed by Associates in Process Improvement (API)–Austin in 1998 from their work in supporting Deming at many of his famous four-day seminars. Often the API improvement advisors were challenged by seminar participants for methods to support the theories that Deming presented. From this challenge the following methods were developed by API:

1. Purpose Statement
2. The Organization Viewed as a System

3. Family of Measures—To measure the effectiveness of the system in accomplishing the purpose of the organization. Often referred to as a "dashboard" or "balanced scorecard."

4. System to Obtain Information—Information focused on matching the *need* in society that the organization served with a focus on customers.

5. Planning—Identifying strategic objectives, improvement efforts, and resources to accomplish the strategy.

6. Managing Individual and Team Efforts—Methods for leaders to ensure that the necessary efforts to design and redesign the system are properly executed and integrated into the organization.

As Maccoby explored these methods he made an observation to the Normans; "What has been developed here are methods to build a foundation for the learning organization." The work was then undertaken to integrate Maccoby's ideas of strategic intelligence with Deming's system of profound knowledge, utilizing the methods for building a foundation for the learning organization.

API has published the methods related to Quality as a Business Strategy (QBS) in their book, *The Improvement Guide: A Practical Approach to Enhancing Organization Performance.* The application of these methods will be discussed in Chapter 10 with applications under the heading of "Building the Foundation for Learning."

While the authors would be flattered to take credit for all the ideas in this book, we are indebted to many who have come before us and have taken the time to help educate us. First and foremost are W. Edwards Deming, Russell Ackoff, and Erich Fromm, who was Maccoby's teacher and colleague.

We also appreciate the contribution of others who have helped us develop the cases and offered criticism of early drafts. They include

Mats Bojestig

Bruce Boles

Alexia Green

Göran Henriks

Jerry Jackson

Brent James

Jonathan Merrell

Fritz Rankin

Jane Roessner

Leslie Schneider

Abby Sears

Tim Scudder

Heather Shearer

David Share

Yedda Trawick

David Wayne

Associates in Process Improvement:

Jerry Langley

Ron Moen

Kevin Nolan

Tom Nolan

Lloyd Provost

Andy Pasternack and Seth Schwartz of Jossey-Bass Wiley gave us helpful advice.

We are grateful to Maria Stroffolino who prepared many drafts of chapters and helped to put this book together.

Endnote

1. National Coalition on Health Care, "Curbing Costs, Improving Care: The Path to an Affordable Health Care Future," 2012.

The Authors

Michael Maccoby is a globally recognized expert on leadership who has consulted to leaders of business, government, universities, and unions in thirty-five countries. He is president of The Maccoby Group in Washington, DC. This is the fourteenth book he has authored or coauthored. His most recent book was *The Leaders We Need: And What Makes Us Follow* (Harvard Business School Press, 2007). He is formerly director of the Program on Technology, Public Policy and Human Development at Harvard (1978–1990) and has taught at a number of universities and the Washington School of Psychiatry. He is currently associate fellow at Oxford's Said Business School. He received a BA and a PhD from Harvard in Social Relations, combining psychology and cultural anthropology. He is a graduate of the Mexican Institute of Psychoanalysis where he studied with Erich Fromm and with him wrote *Social Character in a Mexican Village* (Transaction Publishers, 1996). He is a fellow of the American Psychological Association, the American Anthropological Association, and the National Academy of Public Administration. For his work in Sweden, he was made Commander of the Royal Order of the Polar Star in 2008.

Clifford L. Norman is an internationally recognized consultant on leadership and improvement who has consulted with leaders in business, government, health care, and developed improvement professionals in seventeen countries. He is a coauthor of the first and second editions of *The Improvement Guide—A Practical Approach to Enhancing Organizational Performance*. He received a BA and MA combining police science, business administration, and behavioral science from California State University. He is a senior fellow and improvement advisor with the Institute for Healthcare Improvement (IHI). In 1989, he joined Associates in

Process Improvement (API) after working as a consultant and developing statistical process control materials for Philip Crosby Associates. He is a member of the American Society for Quality and is a certified quality engineer (CQE). With more than thirty years of consulting experience, he is a coowner of Austin API, Inc., and Profound Knowledge Products, Inc.

C. Jane Norman is an internationally recognized consultant on leadership and improvement and has been an executive at Caterpillar, Inc.; ConAgra Inc.; Conrad Company; and OCHIN. With more than thirty years of experience, she has consulted with leaders and developed improvement professionals in manufacturing, food, distribution, technology, software, and health care in twelve countries. She is the coowner of Austin API, Inc., and president of Profound Knowledge Products, Inc., which collaborates with Associates in Process Improvement (API) to develop workshops and virtual learning environments. She is the creator of the accelerated model for improvement (Ami™) methods, developed from the API model for improvement. Ami™ workshops and materials are used worldwide to define and complete improvement projects within one hundred days. She is a certified quality engineer (CQE) with a BA in natural science from St. Ambrose University in Davenport, Iowa, and an MBA from Rollins College in Winter Park, Florida.

Richard Margolies is a health care provider as a clinical psychologist in a psychotherapy practice with high-functioning adults. For over thirty-five years he has also consulted to leaders on developing their leadership and organization. He has worked with businesses and organizations in the private and public sectors, including international organizations and the U.S. Army Corps of Engineers. He is vice president of The Maccoby Group. He has been a research assistant on a number of Michael Maccoby's books, assisted him in the Robert Wood Johnson Foundation funded study of leadership in exemplary health care systems and consulting with two health care organizations. His PhD dissertation was *The Psychoanalytic Meaning of Work*. He and his wife, Cynthia, a clinical psychologist and psychoanalyst, have two children and live in Washington, DC.

PART 1

The Challenge to Health Care Organizations and Creating the Leadership Team

1

INTRODUCTION

From Management Myths
to Strategic Intelligence

Better quality care for more people, improved health, and lower costs. From which source is this statement more likely?

A. A political campaign
B. A well-documented study about a health care organization

Most people will answer "A." Common beliefs and experiences teach us that you can't get more from less. But experiences may be limited, and many common beliefs are myths. We invite you to suspend disbelief while we take you on a tour of **management myths** that make people believe a health care system can't be improved without painful sacrifices. In this book, we will present what we have learned from health care organizations that are improving health care, decreasing per capita costs, and in some cases, improving population health. And we will provide the tools needed to accomplish this seemingly impossible task.

To gain the knowledge needed to master change, it may be necessary to unlearn a number of myths that made sense in a typical bureaucracy but don't work in the kind of learning organizations we'll describe. We use the term *myth* as defined by the *Oxford English Dictionary (OED)*: "a widely held but false belief or idea."[1] Here are just a few myths we will be challenging:

1. The best results are gained by managing by the numbers.
2. People need to be held more accountable.
3. More data are needed to improve management.
4. Incentives will get people to change.
5. Focusing on errors, complaints, and problems will make an organization world class.
6. To get the best people, hire the top 10 percent.
7. Without stretch goals results won't be increased.
8. More people and more money are needed to improve results.
9. To improve quality, it costs more.
10. Leaders are born, not made.
11. People are motivated by a "hierarchy of needs."
12. To motivate people we just need to pay attention to them and be caring bosses.

We have seen the seemingly impossible made possible by health care organizations that challenged these myths and improved quality while cutting costs by achieving the following:

- Less rework (fewer medical errors and readmissions)
- Less waste (better use of facilities, fewer unnecessary tests and procedures)
- Increased collaboration (among health care professionals, staff, patients and their families)

If you aspire to be a leader of change and are willing to question popular theories of management, this book is for you. Many of you have attended lectures or workshops on quality improvement or leadership. But even the best of piecemeal learning will not prepare someone to master change, to transform bureaucracies into learning organizations. We have written this book based on our research and experience of working with health care organizations to provide the understanding and tools to integrate the elements of an effective organization. We are standing on the shoulders of visionary thinkers and have been privileged to learn from them: Russell Ackoff, W. Edwards Deming, and Erich Fromm. We have learned from many others, but these three have contributed especially to our understanding of systems, statistical thinking, theory of knowledge, and psychology.

Improving health care organizations means changing cumbersome bureaucracies into dynamic systems that are patient-focused, cost-effective, and propelled by collaborative learning. This requires culture change, and the first change will be with leaders throughout the organization. No one can do it alone. Leaders need to work together and enlist willing partners and collaborators to achieve these goals.

Knowledge leaders are also needed to network with people outside the organization to bring new ideas and knowledge into the system. A destructive myth that is all too common in many health care organizations is: "We know best." A not-invented-here syndrome rejects thinking from outside the organization and makes life miserable for able knowledge leaders. In one well-known health care organization, they either reject ideas that come from outside the system or, if they adopt an idea, they rebrand it with their own name. They have a habit of not referencing the original author. Learning organizations pride themselves on the ability to learn from many sources and also understand the need to recognize original contributions to their thinking, both from within and outside the organization.

Another commonly believed myth is that physicians will only follow physicians, and as one MD hospital director commented, "When MDs become administrators, they are no longer considered physicians." However, physicians and other health care professionals will follow a leader with the knowledge and personality qualities essential to change bureaucracies into learning organizations. It is a myth that these leaders need to be caring ombudsmen. The leaders we need sometimes pull people outside of their comfort zones. It is also a myth that a good leader has all the answers. The leaders we need are able to make use of the knowledge and learning of all collaborators.

To develop healthy communities, health care organizations must also collaborate with community leaders and public health leaders. In this book, we describe health care organizations that can become models for developing learning communities.

Leaders of learning organizations are different from the administrators of typical health care bureaucracies. Effective administrators are skilled at management functions such as meeting budgets, monitoring functions, and smoothing conflicts. In contrast, a learning organization needs not only good management but also different types of leaders who work interactively to facilitate collaboration, learning, and innovation.

A basic tenet for us is that the person with the relevant knowledge should lead. Some leaders are visionary strategists. Some develop and manage processes and information systems. Some facilitate collaboration at frontline care centers and among all health care providers: physicians, nurses, nurse practitioners, physician assistants, pharmacists, psychologists, social workers, and physical therapists—who also collaborate with technical and administrative staff, and most important, with patients and their families.

Three types fit complementary leadership roles in learning organizations:

- Strategic leaders
- Operational leaders
- Networking leaders

Typically, these leaders have different styles and skills. **Strategic leaders** at the top of organizations are able to design an organization's future and inspire the collaboration needed to implement the vision. In other parts of the organization, they propose new approaches that improve quality. Wherever they are, they are the strategists and architects of change. They need to partner with **operational leaders** who craft the roles and processes that bring the vision to life. The organization also benefits from **networking leaders** who facilitate collaboration between disciplines and organizations to solve complex problems and share learning.

To mold these different types of leaders into an interactive team, the leadership group must articulate a philosophy for the organization. This philosophy should clarify:

- The organization's purpose
- The practical values that are essential for achieving that purpose
- The basis for ethical and moral reasoning used to make decisions
- How results will be defined and measured

At a time when people distrust leaders, it is essential that they can trust a leader's philosophy, that they see a leader sticking to stated values, and that they have no fear of questioning actions that deviate from values that not only support a health care organization's purpose of delivering quality care but also encourage learning, collaboration, and individual initiative.

Effective leadership in knowledge organizations depends not only on the qualities of leaders but also on supporting processes and motivated, qualified people who practice the values essential to achieve the organization's purpose.

This book offers practical methods and tools that can be employed by all types of leaders. However, we have discovered that the skills most needed at the strategic level, what we describe in the framework of **strategic intelligence**, are particularly in short supply. One reason for this is that if they are taught at all, they are taught separately, and not as an interrelated system of skills. Leaders need to recognize the threats and opportunities facing their organizations and then be able to design an organizational vision that takes advantage of this knowledge, and finally, to inspire others to implement the vision.

Strategic intelligence prepares leaders for these interrelated skills, including

- Foresight
- Visioning
- Partnering
- Motivating

These are enabling skills that prepare people to lead productive change.

Strategic intelligence is buttressed by knowledge, not only knowledge of the health care business, but also knowledge about systems, how to deal with variation, the use of statistics for decision making, and the careful testing of theories. These theories are part of what W. Edwards Deming termed **profound knowledge**. Not least, strategic intelligence requires understanding what motivates people, and why they either embrace or resist change. Strategic intelligence combines both soft and hard skills. In the chapters that follow, there are exercises to develop strategic intelligence and profound knowledge. This knowledge challenges a number of management myths.

Make no mistake. Leading change in health care demands commitment, energy, persistence, and knowledge. Health care organizations, particularly hospitals, are among the most complex of organizations. Leaders of health care organizations tend to be overcommitted, responding to demands from all sides. Furthermore, layers of management shield those at the top from the data, views, concerns, and ideas of employees and patients. To make full use of this book, leaders must carve out time for learning. They will model leadership for a learning organization by learning from the experience of all stakeholders—health care providers, employees, patients, and partners. As they make use of what they learn, they will become teachers as well as learners. Then they will be able to lead and drive change.

Plan of the Book

Here is a quick summary of the book's organization. The book is divided into three major parts:

- Part 1: The Challenge to Health Care Organizations and Creating the Leadership Team
  - Chapters 1–4
- Part 2: Strategic Intelligence and Profound Knowledge for Leading
  - Chapters 5–9
- Part 3: Learning from Other Leaders and Creating a Path Forward
  - Chapters 10–11

Part 1: The Challenge to Health Care Organizations and Creating the Leadership Team

Chapter 2 sets the stage for understanding the need for leadership. It describes why and how health care organizations can benefit from change to become learning organizations with these goals:[2]

- Improving quality of care for the patient
- Reducing per capita costs for health care
- Improving population health

These interrelated goals require systemic change in many organizational and medical practices. Some organizations have made great progress toward these goals, and the chapter describes diverse and exemplary learning organizations that are showing the way. Health care organizations are social systems with cultures that differ according to their social, political, and business environments as well as their traditions. Culture, both national and organizational, makes a difference. The people we have worked with in a few countries around the globe are more hierarchical and less collaborative than those we have worked with in Sweden. Physicians at the Mayo and Geisinger Clinics are more collaborative than those we worked with in a number of academic health centers. However, it is a myth that these differences mean that principles of strategic intelligence and profound knowledge cannot be applied to all social systems. Social systems can learn and develop when leaders align innovations with other elements of a system adapted to its environment.

Chapter 3 describes the need for leaders in all parts of an organization to engage participants in the process of change. Leadership, contrasted to management, implies a relationship with followers. Effective leaders of change are hands-on team members, modeling learning and collaboration.

Chapter 4 describes how leaders establish credibility and create trust by formulating, communicating, and practicing a leadership philosophy that includes the organization's purpose, the values essential to achieve that purpose, and a definition of results consistent with the purpose.

Part 2: Strategic Intelligence and Profound Knowledge for Leading

Chapter 5 introduces the concept of strategic intelligence, combining the skills of foresight, visioning, partnering, and motivating. These skills are essential for a leader or leadership team to lead change. They are buttressed by a leadership philosophy plus profound knowledge of organizational systems. *Profound knowledge* includes understanding variation, psychology (personality intelligence), and the theory of knowledge. This knowledge guides the proper use of methods and tools for continual improvement, innovation, and motivation.

Chapter 6 describes how leaders can study and manage their organizations as systems. Russell Ackoff's ideas have been instrumental in our understanding of systems theory and the need for organizations to be viewed as social systems. This starts with understanding the importance of common purpose and the interdependencies among elements of the system. It is a myth that you can improve an organization by improving each of its parts individually. The performance of the system depends more on the interaction of its parts than how the parts perform individually. The chapter describes key systems concepts such as boundaries, feedback loops, constraints, and leverage points. These concepts are useful to develop, test, and implement changes to optimize the system. To manage a system well, it is necessary to measure performance, processes, and results. Another myth is that by holding people accountable, there will be fewer errors. Most errors result from bad processes, not individual mistakes. This leads us to the next chapter.

Chapter 7 describes how statistical thinking aids better and more effective decision making. The chapter describes different ways to understand variation and challenges the myth of managing by the numbers, using dashboards with colored lights to indicate whether or not things are going well. That leads to under- or overreacting without understanding patterns and causes. To understand whether events reflect *common causes* versus *special causes*, graphical methods can be employed to learn from data faster and more effectively. This provides the concepts and methods to understand and manage stable and unstable processes and potential losses due to tampering.

Chapter 8 introduces the concept of personality intelligence, the understanding of the emotional attitudes and values that motivate people at work. Understanding personality intelligence challenges the myths that everyone is motivated by material incentives and that everyone is motivated in the same way. Understanding what motivates people requires that a leader learn psychological concepts and also develop emotional understanding—that is, developing both head and heart. Leaders need to distinguish between behavior shaped by roles and processes contrasted with behavior shaped by motives. We describe changes in the motivating values of professionals raised in the era of a changing family structure and mode of production. Leaders will gain willing collaboration when they understand differences in people's motivation at work and engage their intrinsic motivation by placing them in roles, developing relationships, and clarifying a purpose that connects with their values.

Chapter 9 is about learning, as individuals and organizations. The myth that more information produces greater understanding is challenged. In a time of continual change, leaders need to question and examine their beliefs, assumptions, and knowledge about what makes organizations effective and efficient. They need to develop theories and be open to revising and adapting them in a complex, ever-changing environment. This chapter includes the Model for Improvement (MFI) that provides a road map to ensure that learning is applied. Included in the MFI is the Plan-Do-Study-Act (PDSA) cycle, the engine for improvement that enables the development and trusting of small-scale changes to accelerate learning and the application of knowledge. Also challenged is the myth that people will understand a strategic plan just because it is stated and repeated.

Part 3: Learning from Other Leaders and Creating a Path Forward

Chapter 10 presents case histories of three health care organizations that we recently worked with and studied. These cases illustrate the concepts and methods described in this book. They show how strategically intelligent leaders have improved the quality of care, improved patient health, and lowered costs, and in one case, improved population health.

Chapter 11 presents exercises to turn knowledge into action that gets results. The previous chapters are reviewed with practical exercises to make use of this systems approach to leading change. This chapter provides methods and tools that leaders can use to begin and sustain the process of change.

The authors of this book have studied and worked as advisers to health care organizations in the United States, Canada, United Kingdom, Sweden, and Singapore. It has become clear to us that there is no way health care organizations can avoid changing, but as Deming often remarked: "Survival is not compulsory." New technology, new knowledge, changing values of patients and professionals, government policies, aging of the population in many countries, and rising costs are the factors forcing change. However, change can be either troublesome or productive. Health care organizations can try to react by shrinking service and sacrificing quality or by engaging all employees in creating productive changes, increasing quality of care in a way that reduces costs. They can view their purpose as improving the experience of patients and the health of the communities they serve or as maximizing short-term profit. Which road is taken depends on leadership. We have written this book to provide knowledge, methods, and tools to prepare leaders to choose a productive road, and embark on a sustainable, courageous journey.

KEY TERMS

Management myths
Networking leaders
Operational leaders
Profound knowledge
Strategic intelligence
Strategic leaders

ENDNOTES

1. *Oxford English Dictionary*, 5th ed. (Oxford: Oxford University Press, 2002), 1876.
2. These goals were inspired by W. Edwards Deming's view of a continuum of results. Brent James translated this into a continuum of care moving upstream from patient to population. Donald Berwick instituted these goals as the Triple Aim and they are promoted by the Institute for Healthcare Improvement (IHI) worldwide. Donald M. Berwick, Thomas W. Nolan, and John Whittington, *The Triple Aim: Care, Health, and Cost, Health Affairs* 27, no. 3 (2008), 759–769.

2

WHY AND HOW HEALTH CARE ORGANIZATIONS NEED TO CHANGE

Health care organizations need to change because of avoidable mistakes that harm patients, variability of diagnosis and treatment, and uncontrolled costs.[1] The Institute of Medicine's 2001 report, *Crossing the Quality Chasm*, described these problems.[2] Since that report was published, Don Berwick, one of the report's authors, and others have tirelessly promoted solutions, such as

- Increasing collaboration among clinicians
- Focusing on patient needs
- Giving patients the information essential to share decision making
- Adopting evidence-based treatments
- Driving out waste through targeted improvement efforts

However, these solutions often collide with walls of medical and organizational resistance. This resistance is reinforced by outdated medical protocols and managerial practices, beliefs, and traditional roles that may have served in the past but no longer do so. This resistance stifles the adoption of advances in knowledge, technology, organization, and patient willingness to collaborate in their treatment. It leaves most health care organizations with a **mode of production** and delivery system that is maladapted to our time.

A mode of production describes the way people work in a culture to produce the greatest possible value given the available technology and the knowledge of workers. Based on notable examples from our research and consulting, we show that the mode of production needed for health care organizations requires leaders with different theories and qualities from those that served in the past.

This chapter describes a health care mode of production and delivery system that is able to produce improved health care, reduced per capital costs, and also achieve better health for communities. To improve community health, the focus must be on transforming what is currently sick care into real health care. This implies that organizations not only serve patients (Latin for "those who suffer") but also engage them in maintaining their health and the whole community in preventing illness and improving the quality of life.

Historically, there have been three dominant modes of production in Western societies, characterized by different tools, work roles, relationships and organizations; these are

- Craft-independent
- Industrial-bureaucratic
- Knowledge-interactive

The craft mode is characterized in medicine by the use of hand tools and transferring individual medical skills via master-apprenticeship relationships. The first study of medicine in the Western world is generally acknowledged to have taken place in Greece, where the Greek physician Hippocrates taught in the 5th century BC as the master to his apprentices. The apprenticeship model is still being practiced, renamed as an internship. Traditionally, nursing also used the apprenticeship model with the role of servant to the physician. In 1860, the first school of nursing was established with instruction focused upon the need for hygiene and task competence.

Craftsmen traditionally have belonged to guilds that control entry into professions, rules, and standards. Where medical schools control entry into the medical professions, guilds still exist in the form of societies and associations within each country that control the rules and standards for licensing.

In the industrial-bureaucratic mode of production, workers are placed in formatted roles and are expected to follow rules. Relationships are hierarchical and individual output is measured. Hospitals and most clinics fit this model. Physicians are usually at the top of the hierarchy, with nurses and care technicians at the bottom. But administrators consider themselves the bosses of physicians with the responsibility to ensure conformance to protocol. Their role includes the ability to hire and fire personnel. However, physicians generally decide the rules and diagnosis and treatment protocols they will follow, and if threatened, they can leave a hospital, taking their patients with them. Because they are trained in the craftsman model, many believe they should make the rules and define their own roles. This creates an informal hierarchy above the administrator who formally oversees protocol conformance. When physicians become employees, their productivity is measured by how many patients they see each working day. Productivity of administrators is measured according to variance of the budget and control of costs, balanced against the retention of physicians. Productivity of nurses can generally be measured by how many patients a nurse is responsible for. In general, the lower the hierarchy, the more patients and tasks for which the role is responsible.

Hospitals have benefitted by learning from industrial production systems, particularly process improvement through simplification and standardization of protocol, procedures, and sharing of information (see Chapters 6 and 7). Making it easy to do the right thing and hard to do the wrong thing shifts efforts away from blaming individuals working in a poorly designed system to developing and managing a strategically aligned systemwide improvement effort. However, within the framework of an industrial mode of production, some physicians remain fixated in the craft mode they were taught in medical school. They resist positive efforts to reduce variation inpatient outcomes, terming them "cookbook medicine" which does not consider unique patient needs. To be sure, medicine is still an art based on science and the qualities of a physician. Some doctors are better diagnosticians and performers than others. But for many cases there are clear pathways for treatment.

Physicians resent becoming employees in a bureaucracy, where they become "providers" or managers who are engaged more in monitoring than mentoring and must focus on business profitability rather than solely on the well-being of patients.

When medicine was a craft, the patient was usually the payer. When health care is delivered in an impersonal production system, focus on the patient is weakened by the need to serve the new payers: insurance companies, Medicare and Medicaid, or other government agencies. When payment is based on performing a formatted task or completing a number of appointments, a health care provider is less able to take account of a patient's complexities. Ten- to fifteen-minute appointments leave little time for collaboration, understanding, and building knowledge with the patient. Measures of physician productivity are designed to fit the payers' requirements (billing codes) and the organization's budget.[3]

In addition, when patients do not have an ongoing relationship with a particular healer, whether it is a physician, psychologist, nurse practitioner, or physical therapist, but are sent to different providers, the professional is less likely to know the patient's personality and history. The lack of an ongoing relationship limits the positive transference that facilitates healing, and it becomes more difficult to gain collaboration from patients, families, and their support units.

The age of information technology with the arrival of computers, electronic medical records (EMR), and the Internet has catapulted medicine toward the knowledge-interactive mode of production. Elements of this model have infiltrated some aspects of the industrial-bureaucratic mode of production through the technology of diagnostic tools that require trained technicians to interpret the results and consult with physicians. Information technology can facilitate continual learning to increase the ability of cross-functional and interdisciplinary teams to interact and collaborate with stakeholders to innovate and improve. Table 2.1 summarizes the elements of the three modes of production. Maccoby constructed the table, with the help of Paul Griner and Roger Bulger, both visionary physician leaders. The table and the need to transform health care organizations to the knowledge-interactive mode has been affirmed by leaders at Intermountain Healthcare, Mayo Clinic, Kaiser Permanente, Geisinger Clinic, and Vanderbilt University Medical Center among others.

The danger for the future of health care is that the traditional craft-independent mode of production continues to transition to the industrial-bureaucratic mode, which further reinforces the separation of physicians, nurses, technicians, and other health care professionals into silos of knowledge, where workers perform independently in a health care factory. Alternatively, the knowledge-interactive mode of production begins with a patient focus on the part of health care professionals that empowers them to match care to individual patient need, resulting

Table 2.1 Modes of Production in Health Care

	Craft-Independent	Industrial-Bureaucratic	Knowledge-Interactive
Medical Diagnostic Tools	• Physical examination • Patient history • Modern age: Same as industrial and knowledge	• Mechanical: stethoscope, blood pressure monitor • Electro: X-ray, EKG, MRI, ultrasound • Chemical: blood tests, DNA	• Same as craft and industrial plus: • Information and social technology
Roles	• Individual • Master-apprentice	• Formal job description	• Interdependent • Role descriptions • Flexibility guided by purpose and values
Responsibilities	• Multiple (as needed)	• As defined by job description	• Implement defined processes • Improve self and processes, products, and services
Relationships	• Master-apprentice	• Hierarchical • Addition of administrator	• Collaborative
Relationship with Patient	• Physician authority • Submissive-trusting	• Provider • Customer	• Teacher-collaborator • Learner-collaborator
Business Model	• Personal relationships • Reputation	• Price • Scale • Service	• Coproduction • Prevention • Health improvement
Model of Care	• Biomedical	• Biomedical	• Biopsychosocial • Epidemiological
Leadership Model	• Master-apprentice • Mentor • Ombudsman	• Manager • Monitor	• Strategic • Operational • Networking • Person with knowledge leads
Values	• Caring • Personal trust • Expertise	• Expertise • Profitability • Service	• Caring • Trust—both ways • Collaborative expertise • Quality • Innovation
Knowledge	• Resides within individuals	• Resides within departmental silos and individuals	• Shared learning from experience and through testing of ideas
Organization	• Workshop-guild • Private practice	• Bureaucracy • Hospitals/clinics	• Learning • Integrated patient-focused care

in better care and lower overall costs. We have studied and advised a few health care organizations that are attempting to create **learning organizations** that employ a knowledge-interactive mode of production. We believe these examples of organizations and leadership can be extremely useful to others who are striving to improve the delivery, cost and quality of health care, and ultimately the health of their communities.

The Purpose of the Preliminary Research

The purpose of the study that partly informs this chapter was to understand the leadership visions and implementation strategies of fifteen health care organizations and academic health centers selected by a panel of distinguished medical and nursing leaders to be among the best in the United States.[4] The leadership competencies and tools required to transform these organizations to adapt to new economic, technological, and social conditions were explored by interviewing a sample of key medical and administrative leaders in each of these organizations. Added to this study, which was carried out in 2000, is the continuing experience of the authors as consultants to health care organizations in the United States, Canada, United Kingdom, Sweden, and Singapore that are striving to become learning organizations. Three of these organizations are described in Chapter 10.

The Model of Change

Three principles have emerged from our research and consulting:

1. A health care learning organization should be patient-focused.
2. Patient knowledge, advocacy, and shared decision making are enhanced by information technology and social media. They can result in more productive relationships between patients and providers.
3. Health care organizations are social systems made up of people with different values and purposes. Leadership is needed to create common values and purpose.

The first principle is that in a patient-focused health care system, health care providers should be able to develop trusting relationships with their patients. Without this patient focus and freedom from bureaucratic constraints that impede collaboration and innovation, the most qualified young people will go into other professions where they can better realize their potential.

The second principle recognizes the increasing impact of an informed public. Patients and their families are researching medical conditions and options via the Internet and demanding to review and understand them with health care professionals. Patients of the past who did not question a physician's knowledge and judgment are being replaced by informed computer-savvy people who are using the Internet for research and becoming patient advocates for their parents, children, and for themselves. The challenging, collaborative patient can be found in the Internet world of chats, blogs, and sites such as e-patient. com. These active patients can either help improve the quality and cost of care or they can increase costs by demanding unnecessary tests and care. Which alternative prevails depends in large part on the ability of health care professionals to develop learning relationships with patients and their families. It also depends on the ability of patients to access information about the quality of care delivered by providers and hospitals.

The third principle is that to improve health care organizations, they must be recognized and understood as social systems made up of people with their own values and purposes. A social system can't be changed just by installing new technology and processes. Leaders must align processes with practical values and motivate competent people to achieve the organization's purpose.

At the beginning of the research project, we carried out in-depth interviews with physician leaders in an effort to understand their shared values or *social character*, a concept discussed in Chapter 8. What kind of a health system did they consider ideal? They expressed serious concerns about the deterioration of the physician's professional freedom and ability to develop relationships of trust with patients. However, although freedom for physicians to be patient-focused can enhance relationships with their patients, colleagues, and even their organizations, the physician leaders believed that autonomy in medical decision making should be encouraged when the answers are known, based on evidence of what treatment works best. Since these interviews took place, nurses, psychologists, and other health care professionals have increasingly challenged the dominant role of physicians in certain clinical and leadership roles.

Changing Modes of Production in Health Care

In the study of health care organizations selected by the panel of experts, health care was viewed from an anthropological perspective, focusing on the changing mode of production. A mode of production refers not only to the use of tools. It describes a productive system of values, beliefs, rules, and relationships that may change over time due to new technology, knowledge, and innovation. For example, agriculture was produced by a craft-family-farm mode of production in 1840 when over 70 percent of the U.S. workforce tilled the soil using traditional methods. Today, less then 2 percent of the American workforce produces enough food to feed a much larger U.S. population and to export the surplus abroad. Agriculture in America is highly mechanized and uses biochemical technology. Large farms are run by agribusinesses. Animals are raised in factories. The mode of production, including work roles and relationships, has been transformed into industrial and knowledge modes. The independent craft farmers fought the change as long as they could, but relatively few of them remain in business.

Health Care in Learning Organizations

Advanced organizational thinking emerging from most effective professional service companies provides elements of a health care mode of production and delivery system that focuses on the health of individual patients and improves outcomes while lowering costs. This alternative enables physicians and other providers to be creative, yet it retains the best qualities of the craft tradition. In manufacturing or industrial service organizations, productivity depends essentially on the organization's people, processes, practices, and how these are orchestrated into a system that achieves its purpose. The producer alone can control productivity. In professional services, as in the most advanced knowledge industries, productivity depends on both producer and client, on coproduction and continual learning. The lawyer or accountant's productivity rises when the clients learn to keep good records and follow productive practices. IBM helps a business customer improve productivity by customizing its products and services to the customer's needs. This is also the case for health care, most clearly with chronic conditions. When patients manage their own conditions, control their diets and exercise, keep their own records, and medicate themselves, their health improves and medical costs are lowered. Furthermore, as patients gain easier access to medical information on the Internet, opportunities increase for provider-patient partnering to improve patient health and keep costs in check. But unless they are informed and engaged, patients will not take responsibility for their care, medication, healthy diet, and exercise.

Both a craft and a bureaucratic health care organization can deliver care. But only a collaboration between providers and patients in a learning organization can produce health. Learning can be facilitated among patients and their families for treatment of chronic conditions such as diabetes, asthma, obesity, and depression. Prevention and management does not depend just on costly visits to physicians. Some health care learning organizations, like that of Jönköping in Sweden described in Chapter 10, organize and facilitate patient support groups that meet regularly to educate and encourage patients to care for themselves. For health care organizations to make full use of informatics and quality processes, they must become learning organizations within a knowledge-interactive mode of production. As a learning organization, a health care organization has several defining attributes:

- Developed as a social system (see Chapters 5 and 6) where all the parts interact to achieve the purpose of serving patients

  - Designing and redesigning the system of delivering care decreases per capita cost while maintaining or improving patient outcomes

- Learning from practice is widely shared and used for innovation and improvement

  - Partners with suppliers, client organizations, and community organizations
  - Providers collaborate across disciplines, with patients and their families

- Learning is used to inform the community, aid in the prevention of illness, and improve population health

In a learning organization, providers act to further organizational purpose, not in response to bureaucratic command and control, but because they have internalized the purpose and share its values. They do not see a contradiction between their autonomy and the organization's goals. For example, physicians will be convinced that by improving the quality of information and the care delivery system, they will benefit their patients, the organization, and the community and reduce the total cost of health care.

Such a system needs information technology to aid decision making. People should not be dependent on a health care delivery system to make healthy choices or understand when they should seek a health care professional's help. And when they become patients, they deserve an experience that is safe, free of hassles, and responsive to their individual needs. Thus, the system requires both advanced integrated organizational design informatics, and committed, informed professionals—nurses, psychologists, physical therapists, social workers, administrators, and technicians as well as physicians. It requires electronic medical records available to all the patient's providers. Encouragement, training, and easy access to useful information for the patient, patient advocates, and their support system will continue to challenge and improve the system.

Furthermore, the ideal health system will challenge all health care professionals to work together to improve the health of a community. This requires an expansion of the care model from a purely biomedical craft focus to a biopsychosocial and epidemiological ecosystem focus. It will call for a different kind of medical education such as the type pioneered by the University of Rochester Medical School where medical students learn to collaborate with other providers and with their patients.

Finally, to build the foundation of the learning organization requires methods. Chapter 10 will present case studies from our clients where the following methods have been utilized to build the foundation of the learning organization:

1. *Purpose:* Use of a purpose statement that communicates the aim of the organization and the practical values necessary to accomplish this aim and serve customers, patients, and their families. This purpose is driven by the leadership philosophy of the organization.
2. *Viewing the organization as a system:* A model of the organization that describes how work is actually accomplished by a linkage of processes.
3. *Family of measures:* Use of the key measures of the organization that informs stakeholders how well the organization is meeting its purpose. Commonly referred to as a dashboard or balanced scorecard.

4. *Sources of information for learning:* A system to ensure that information is collected from inside and outside the organization with a focus on patients, families, and customers.
5. *Strategic planning:* Plans to improve and operate to ensure that the idealized vision of the future is achieved.
6. *Managing individual and team efforts:* Defining the role of leaders to ensure that change efforts are identified, resourced, and executed.

Leadership for Learning

Such a system requires a leadership theory and skills different from either the craft or industrial-bureaucratic modes of production. Maccoby first proposed this typology of modes of production in 1998 at the annual meeting of the Association of Academic Health Centers. It was well received by the attending CEOs and became the leading chapter in the Association's publication *Creating the Future*.[5] In 1999, Maccoby led a workshop with leaders of academic health centers to determine the gaps between the practices of a learning organization and current practice, via a gap survey. In our consulting, we have continued to give health care leaders questionnaires that measure these gaps.

In 1999, the major gaps between the ideal and current practice indicated by leaders of health care centers were the following:

- **Patient service as the highest priority was an ideal universally stated but seldom achieved.** We found this gap at all academic health care centers studied, with the exception of the Mayo Clinic. (The gap was also small at Intermountain Health Care (IHC), the Geisinger Clinic, and Kaiser Permanente in Oakland, California.)
- **Utilization management is a gap shared by all physicians that reflects the craft mode of production.** There is significant variability in the way the same presenting problem is treated by different physicians in health care organizations.
- **Information systems support physician decision making.** This gap is now being addressed by all the health care organizations we studied. However, the approaches vary. The danger for organizations is that new information systems are not aligned with a learning culture but rather are focused on payment systems. (A notable positive model has been developed at Vanderbilt University Medical Center.)

In a learning organization, system performance is evaluated regularly as it contributes or deters individual performance. Each person is expected to share knowledge. Everyone teaches and the system learns.

- **Leaders develop relationships of trust.** A number of factors cause the trust gap. As health care leaders pressure their organizations to cut costs in the name of improved performance, distrust can increase. A large part of the problem reflects a lack of dialogue between leaders and their organizations about the need for change and how best to achieve it. As we discuss in Chapter 4, leaders need to communicate a philosophy including purpose, the values essential to achieve that purpose, and how results will be measured. There must be transparency about the flow of money. By viewing the organization as a system with a purpose that needs continuous improvement, individuals will be able to stop the blame game and focus on improving the system. They will be able to focus on specific outcomes and what it takes to develop a financially secure organization. To achieve collaboration and facilitate learning with patients and providers, health care organizations need leaders who model a collaborative, learning environment within the organization. Transformation of an organization takes time, patience, and constancy of purpose, particularly from the executive leadership team and their governing board.

- **Leaders communicate a vision.** The professionals we have interviewed want to know what their organization is trying to become and how they fit in this vision. A vision statement such as "we will be the best health care organization" or "we will be a model for innovation" is no substitute for a systemic vision of the organization, its purpose, and the way people will work together. Given the uncertainty in health care, people at all levels of the organization want leaders to set a clear course, explain the logic underlying it, and help them to understand the meaning of change for them.

The Human Side of Change

We found that the culture of health care organizations and social character of physicians play a key role in facilitating or impeding change. Based on social character interviews and surveys of senior physicians and graduating physicians, we found a dominant value constellation or shared social character. Most physicians fit a type we termed *expert-helper*. The dominant value for the expert is mastery, including the need for achievement. The expert's sense of self-esteem and employment security is achieved by gaining status and professional respect. Experts find pleasure at work in their craftsmanship and recognition by their peers and superiors. They have a strong need for autonomy. At their best, experts stand for high standards of service and scientifically proven knowledge. They value professionalism, a term with roots in the Calvinist concept of professing a calling to serve. At their worst, their obsessive qualities make experts inflexible know-it-alls.

The education of physicians trains them to fit into a system of master and apprentice, where knowledge is based on experience, at a time when knowledge is quickly out of date and competence depends on continual learning. Thus, the expert's character can be a major roadblock to change. Experts want to control their activities. They view the empowerment of others as loss of control. This has been a complaint heard repeatedly from nurses and administrators.

Physician experts tend to see their organizations as service functions and do not appreciate the added value of an organization over what they do as individuals. Physicians, like other experts, relate best with mentors, peers, or younger high-potential apprentices who share their values.

Approach to Service

The *Oxford English Dictionary* defines *expert* as "experienced" and "trained by practice or experience; skilled or skillful."[6] Expert comes from the Latin "expertus," meaning tried, experienced. The expert's awards and diplomas are typically displayed to attest to experience and achievement. The physician experts interviewed see the meaning of their work not only in the excellence of their performance, but also in helping people.

Notably, some of the most innovative physician leaders we interviewed had a somewhat different social character, with a focus on creating a great organization. These leaders were typically productive narcissists, the visionary type of personality described by Sigmund Freud as not impressed by the status quo but "especially suited to act as a support for others, to take on the role of leaders, and to give a fresh stimulus to cultural development or damage the established state of affairs."[7] While the craft experts see health care organizations as little more than a support for their craftwork, innovative leaders understand that effective organizations are essential to achieve the goal of better health care in a cost-effective manner. This difference in thinking about the organization can cause a profound disconnection between leaders and physicians.

Although we have not done these interviews with a sample of nurses, Cliff and Jane Norman have observed from the responses of nurses to the SDI questionnaire (see Chapter 8 for a description of this questionnaire) that their dominant motivation at work is helping people. This finding supports testimony by nurses that conflicts with physicians occur when nurses judge that a physician is not responding to their concerns about a patient's needs. And nurses often complain that physicians do not respect their judgment.

The Role of Culture

In most medical schools, physicians are selected and trained to be autonomous craftsmen. There is little teaching about interdependence, leadership, or the importance of organization. Physicians are not trained to look at work from the viewpoint of nurses, psychologists, pharmacists, technicians, or even patients. The image of the independent decision maker that may have made the field attractive to them is reinforced by their education. Expert physicians are comfortable within a craft mode of production. Their ideal organization is their own craft shop or possibly a partnership.

With some frustration, the physician can also fit into the semifeudal academic health center. In this organization, the vice president for the medical center takes a role like that of a feudal lord and the chairs become barons who determine which of the physician vassals are most favored. To carry the analogy further, the academic specialists are often viewed by the local MDs (LMDs) or primary care physicians as superior beings who demand tribute and referrals but show little or no respect to the peasant-like LMDs.

Many of the faculty members interviewed seek to maintain their autonomy through research grants that allow them to set up their own shops. They can justify being part of an academic organization for the prestige it provides them as professors. Because independence, prestige, and promotions depend on research grants and publications, service to patients is not their first priority. Furthermore, this system rewards individuals and not collaborative groups.

We also found a culture clash between physicians and hospital administrations. In a sense, this is a conflict between the craft logic of individual authority, self-generated revenue, personal style of care, and being the patient's advocate as opposed to the bureaucratic logic of centralized administration, financial controls, standardized procedures, and rules based on principles of fairness. This clash can at least be partly resolved by developing the kind of transparent learning culture described more fully in later chapters.

The typical pattern of leading academic health centers results in a corrosive hierarchy of status. The full-time clinicians feel slighted and also believe that many medical researchers do not spend enough time with patients to maintain their competence. We often heard the view that individual physicians could no longer sustain the triple ideal of teaching, research, and practice. There was not total agreement about this, however, and some physicians appeared successful at combining the three functions.

The Mayo Model

An exception to the prevailing pattern is the group practice culture, most notably as developed by the Mayo Clinic. At Mayo, the patient comes first. Research and teaching are important but secondary, and research is aimed at improving clinical outcomes. Furthermore, specialists cooperate across disciplines in a way seldom seen in other academic health centers where patients with medical problems that cross disciplines also lack the benefit of the coordinating team of Mayo physicians. Mayo doctors are salaried and all departments are treated as cost centers. Physicians can take as much time with patients as they consider necessary. And administrators at Mayo see their role as serving physicians rather than struggling with them about costs. The nurses at St. Francis Hospital in Rochester, Minnesota, feel respected as colleagues, not subordinates. There is a smaller trust gap at Mayo than in any of the other academic health centers we studied.

The Mayo Value Creation System is a process that Mayo authors write "has been demonstrated to improve the quality of patient care while reducing costs and increasing productivity."[8] Mayo demonstrates how to create a learning organization that engages administrators and clinicians in a shared purpose. "There is no trade-off between improving quality and decreasing cost," the Mayo authors report. "In fact, when viewed from the whole of a balanced portfolio of value creation, they occur concurrently if undertaken with a disciplined and balanced systems engineering approach while keeping the best interests of the patient in mind."[9]

The natural question we asked ourselves is whether the Mayo Clinic and other group practices built on the Mayo model, such as Geisinger, Cleveland Clinic, and Dartmouth-Hitchcock, attract physicians with a different, more cooperative social character or, alternatively, whether the different cultures and incentives shape the values of physicians. Mayo favors hiring physicians who have been socialized in the culture as medical students and residents. As we have not done a longitudinal study of physicians starting with their choice of a place to work or even a choice of residencies, our answer to the question remains somewhat speculative.

However, we were able to interview over 120 physicians and administrators from an academic health center and a clinic modeled after Mayo, at a time when the two organizations were trying unsuccessfully to merge. In the clash of cultures, we also observed a difference in the values that were reinforced by the two cultures.

Maccoby and Margolies were hired by the leadership of the two organizations to help develop a common culture based largely on the learning model. In workshops attended by physicians from the two cultures, participants filled out gap questionnaires and the results showed there was strong support for this model. On the gap questionnaires (see Chapter 11 for an example), both physicians and administrators indicated that the elements of the model were important for improving their organizations. However, the leadership groups including some departmental chairs of the two organizations saw themselves and their counterparts in different ways that emphasized their own virtues and the other's supposed defects.

Groups of department chairs from the two organizations were asked to agree on the qualities they believed described themselves and those that described the other organization. The academic chairs described themselves as open to new ideas, participants in decision making who were able to question authority. They saw themselves as entrepreneurial capitalists. They described the clinic physicians as employees of a centralized, bureaucratic collective: rule-driven conformists who did not question authority. The clinic chairs saw themselves as placing the highest value on patient service in contrast to the faculty physicians who put their publications before their patients. They stated that since they received a fixed salary, financial incentives did not distort their clinical practice. They could take as much time as needed with each patient. They contrasted their cooperative interdependence with their characterization of the faculty physicians as individualistic and careerist. They affirmed their respect for LMDs and the primary-tertiary care relationship and accused the faculty specialists of being arrogant, controlling, and self-serving.

These stereotypes distorted the chairs' views of each other. For example, the faculty chairs were convinced that their results were better than those of the clinic. That may have been true for some specialties. However, they were unaware that the clinics' coronary artery bypass (CABG) results were better than theirs and achieved at a lower cost.

How different were the physicians in these two cultures? If you moved any of them from one culture to another, would their behavior change? In our view some chairs strongly expressed the cultural values of their organizations while others were less polarized. After this meeting, Maccoby and Margolies facilitated a discussion with the Department of Medicine of both groups. The stereotypes were discussed, and the participants agreed to try to create a common culture, using the model of a learning organization. The younger physicians were most clearly in favor of close cooperation and shared leadership. The older ones agreed to make a sincere attempt. They recognized that this required strong leadership to resolve conflict and affirm the common vision. The attempt to create a common culture was short-circuited when top leadership could not work together, and the boards of directors voted to dissolve the merger.

SUMMARY

No longer will patients passively wait for the health care community to tell them what to do. Their expectations are challenging the existing health care delivery systems, health care professionals, and information systems. The ability of patients to evaluate their conditions, care, and options via the Internet challenges traditional relationships, craft- and production-oriented health care systems, and their providers. Partnering and the integration of informed patients and patient advocates into the delivery system will differentiate health care organizations as they transform into the interactive health care learning environment of the future.

Physicians have run clinics or their own medical offices. Yet their education does not include courses to help them manage and improve complex health care organizations, much less lead others to do so. If physicians and nurses are to lead learning organizations, they must develop new skills and knowledge.

There is resistance to change, particularly from physicians whose social character and training support the craft mode of production. Unless the education of physicians focuses on developing the values and competencies for a learning organization, resistance will continue to impede positive change. However, we met many younger physicians with a more interactive social character who respond in a more positive way to a learning organization (see Chapter 8).

Nurses are often the behind-the-scenes leaders within clinics, wards, and offices, running the business and managing patient care. They work in partnership with physicians, specialists, administrators, and other nurses. Many times they defer to the physician or manager in charge. They generally choose not to lead, even when they understand better than formal authority figures the personalities and viewpoints of physicians, nurses, and other professionals and patients. They tend to defer to the physician as the leader. They need to develop leadership competence and confidence. Leadership in learning organizations should be based on knowledge and leadership qualities, not professional affiliation. All health care workers should be respected for their distinctive competences.

Health care organizations are cultures or social systems that have purposes and are composed of people who must be motivated to achieve these purposes. These cultures differ according to their social, political, and business environments and traditions as well as their missions. They select and socialize different values in their key members. Social systems will learn and develop only when leaders align innovations with other elements of the system. Otherwise, new ideas and approaches will be limited, distorted, or totally rejected. The good news is that some of the leaders of health care organizations are becoming aware of what is required to transform their systems, and they are providing models that others can learn from, but not necessarily copy. Adaptation and testing to fit local circumstances are critical to successful implementation.

Leaders of some of the best health care organizations in the United States, Canada, United Kingdom, Sweden, and other countries strongly affirm the need to move to the learning mode of production. Elements of the learning mode are emerging in some of these organizations, but creating a learning organization requires leadership and continual development.

Policymakers should understand that solving the problems of health care delivery is not just a matter of adopting new policies and incentives, but rather of transforming a craft mode of production in a way that incorporates the best craft values into more productive, interactive learning organizations.

Leaders for health care organizations should be selected not because they are distinguished experts, but because they demonstrate strategic intelligence and understand the logic of business, quality, and leadership. They must gain the informed support of their boards, recognizing that even positive change will provoke resistance.

The next chapter will elaborate on the kinds of leaders needed to change health care organizations.

KEY TERMS

Learning organization

Mode of production

EXERCISES

1. Consider the attributes of the Modes of Production in Health Care in Table 2.1. Which best describes your organization:
   - Craft-independent?
   - Industrial-bureaucratic?
   - Knowledge-interactive?

2. Consider your organization:
   - Is it a learning organization as defined by the attributes in this chapter? If not, do you believe it needs to become a learning organization?
   - If yes, why is this necessary? Think about what needs to change relative to the defined attributes.
   - Share this chapter with key leaders in your organization and discuss the reasons why you need to become a learning organization.

ENDNOTES

1. Some of the research behind this chapter was funded by the Robert Wood Johnson Foundation. Maccoby, the lead investigator, was assisted by Richard Margolies, Barbara Lenkerd, George Casey, and Doug Wilson. Valuable counsel was given by an advisory committee including (their then positions): Polly Banish, PhD, RN, FAAN, Executive Director, American Association of Colleges of Nursing; Roger Bulger, MD, President, Association of Academic Health Centers; Paul Griner, MD, former President, American College of Physicians and Vice President and Director, Center for the Assessment and Management of Change in Academic Medicine, Association of American Medical Colleges; Federico Ortiz Quesada, MD, Director, International Relations, Mexican Ministry of Health; Stan Pappelbaum, MD, former CEO, Scripps Health; Richard Riegelman, MD, MPH, PhD, Dean, School of Public Health and Health Services, George Washington University; Henry Simmons, MD, President, National Leadership Coalition on Health Care.

2. Institute of Medicine, *Crossing the Quality Chasm: A New Health System for the 21st Century* (Washington, DC: National Academy Press, 2001).

3. Most electronic medical records (EPIC, NextGen, Bridgefront, and so on) were designed first around billing needs (reimbursement from Medicare or Medicaid and their sliding scales), rather than care needs. More and more programs external or secondary are now being developed (solutions) to allow empanelment and patient population management.

4. Our views of the need to transform health care organizations are based both on study trips taken by Maccoby and Margolies, and consulting on change by Maccoby and Margolies and by Cliff and Jane Norman. We made study trips to the University of Rochester Medical Center, Intermountain Health Care, Penn State, Geisinger, Aetna U.S. Health Care Southeastern Region, University of Michigan Medical Center, Shands-University of Florida (Margolies with Barbara Lenkerd), and Mayo Clinic at Rochester, Minnesota, Mayo Clinic at Scottsdale, Arizona, Vanderbilt University Medical Center, and Kaiser Permanente in Oakland, California. Maccoby consulted to the University of Georgetown Medical Center, Scripps Health, Penn State Medical Center, and Geisinger Clinic (with Margolies). The Normans have consulted with SingHealth, Cherokee Nation, CareOregon, OCHIN, NHS in the United Kingdom, Jönköping County Council in Sweden, Canadian Healthcare in the provinces of Ontario, British Columbia, and Alberta.

5. Clyde H. Evans and Elaine R. Rubin (eds.), *Creating the Future: Innovative Programs and Structures in Academic Health Centers* (Washington, DC: Association of Academic Health Centers, 1999).

6. *Oxford English Dictionary*, 5th ed. (Oxford: Oxford University Press, 2002), 895.

7. Michael Maccoby, *Narcissistic Leaders: Who Succeeds and Who Fails* (Boston: Harvard Business School Press, 2007).

8. Stephen J. Swenson, MD, James Dilling, BSIE, CMPE, C. Michael Harper Jr., MD, and John H. Noseworthy, MD, "The Mayo Clinic Value Creation System," *American Journal of Medical Quality* 27, no.1 (Jan/Feb 2012), 58–65.

9. Ibid.

3

LEADING HEALTH CARE CHANGE

Without effective **leaders**, health care organizations will not become learning organizations. Leaders are needed to protect the best qualities of caring and service found in the craft tradition of medicine and nursing and also build on them to establish new ways of working. With the active participation of staff, leaders are needed to continuously improve patient safety and outcomes, reduce unnecessary costs, enhance patients' experience of service, and improve population health. Above all, leaders are needed to encourage the doubters, to infuse the belief that the people can create the organization's future.

Some health care organizations do conceive of their purpose as developing a continuum of care from the patient upstream to improving the health of the community, adopting the **Triple Aim** of better patient outcomes, reduced per capita cost, and improved population health. An example is the University of Rochester Medical Center (URMC), which developed the biopsychosocial model of medicine. In that tradition, URMC studied the epidemiological data in its community to discover ways to prevent illness and improve health. Subsequently, Rochester staff taught asthmatics in the community how to clean their homes of allergens; this understanding was made part of medical education. Another example, described in Chapter 10, is the Jönköping community, a health care organization that keeps learning and engaging the community to prevent illness and improve health.

Leaders of health care organizations cannot expect that change will come about by administering a stable organization, managing anonymously by rules, using carrots and sticks. They will not change organizations by making inspiring speeches and expecting others to do the work. Effective leaders of change are visible and known by staff as learners who are also teachers. They need to be trained for **leadership** as well as for business. As described in subsequent chapters, this training should include how leaders employ profound knowledge to guide and bring about fundamental change.

What is *leadership*? Leaders are people others follow. If no one follows you, you are not a leader. If you have followers, you are a leader. Leadership is a relationship. Good leadership means people willingly follow a leader who is working to further the common good, the well-being of all stakeholders. Good leaders make followers into collaborators. Leadership implies a relationship that cannot be handed off to anyone else. In contrast, **management** is a collection of functions. Management has to do with measurements, monitoring, HR, supply functions, and the implementation of service delivery necessary for operations. Many management functions do not require managers as teams can share these functions, even rotate them within a team, and some can be automated. Both leadership and management are necessary for the success of organizations. All managers should be leaders, and in fact, most can be developed for leadership roles. As the Institute of Medicine recommends, a continuously learning health care system requires "broad leadership."[1]

However, exceptional leadership is needed to transform an organization from a bureaucracy to a learning organization. Strategic leaders are needed to assess the forces shaping the market and society, to create a vision of how the organization can succeed in the future and a strategy to get there. Once the vision is defined, through a leadership-driven process, leaders need to motivate a diverse staff to work together for that desired future. This requires that leaders build trust between themselves and disciplines and groups that may be in tension with each other about priorities, investments, and roles. No leader can achieve these goals all alone. They need to partner and interact with other leaders who complement their competencies.

Because leadership is a relationship, it cannot, unlike management functions, be delegated, assigned, or transferred. Leaders who are followed for the clarity of their thinking, their dedication to values, and the relationship they have built with others cannot hand this relationship off to anyone else. Because leadership cannot be given away, the question arises: why do people follow a leader? Do they follow because they want to or because they have to? In other words, is it because they trust or fear the leader? Today's workforce of professionals, technicians, and knowledge workers want leaders who seek empowered collaborators, not blind followers. These knowledge workers want to share a common purpose with a leader who is empowering them to be effective in their work.

Leaders in learning organizations clarify an organizational purpose that people find inspiring and can envisage their role in achieving it. These leaders understand the values that motivate people in their work and place them in roles that connect with those values. Part of creating trust is **transparency** about costs, revenues, and investments. With financial transparency, everyone can be assured that resources are used productively. Brent James, the head of informatics at Intermountain Health Care, also defines transparency as giving care providers easy access to all the information they need to make informed decisions about patient care. With this information infrastructure, caregivers can become empowered collaborators.

Leaders for change are needed throughout the organization, not just at the top. We have observed that high-performing knowledge-based organizations require an *interdependent leadership system* with three different types of leadership:

- Strategic
- Operational
- Network

Strategic leaders define purpose and vision, aligning people, processes, and practical values so that they support and further the organization's purpose. Although these leaders may not have all the qualities of strategic intelligence, which will be examined in Chapter 5, they partner with others so that these qualities exist among members of their leadership team. Strategic leaders recognize that change stirs up resistance; therefore, these leaders educate all stakeholders to make them allies. For example, at Kaiser Permanente David Lawrence, the CEO, gained union collaboration and educated the board about the need for change. If board members are not educated about change, they can undermine a change leader. At one large health care organization we worked with, a board member who was grateful for his prior treatment by a physician in the organization led a board vote to veto change, because that physician had lobbied him against the creative CEO who wanted to eliminate the lucrative private deals some physicians enjoyed. The CEO had failed to educate his board about these practices and how they increased unnecessary costs.

Operational leaders focus on making the operations function efficiently and effectively. They may lead operating teams, emergency rooms, or administrative functions. For example, William Stead, a physician and professor at Vanderbilt Medical Center and a visionary operational leader, built a department of informatics, because he saw the future role it could play in enhancing outcome quality, safety, and service delivery. Over time, the Department of Informatics worked with staff across the organization to interactively design an IT system to deliver better health care. Patients were able to manage their chronic conditions and report to their doctors via the Internet. The department also developed IT products for community health such as their CD-ROM for parents and teachers about how to socialize aggressive children. This example shows the interaction of strategic and operational leaders in developing new processes and products to improve service outcomes as well as enhancing the health of the population.

Network leaders connect people across disciplines, organizational departments, and regions. They create trust and build the bridges required to make groups into collaborative teams. Network leaders may be physicians who ensure that patients receive the best possible treatment, such as the internists at Mayo who take charge of a patient and make sure all specialists work together on the case. They may be nurses and administrators who lead the kind of improvement teams described in Chapters 6 and 7 and in the cases reported in Chapter 10. Ideally, operational leaders also have qualities of network leaders. However, network leaders are most effective when they do not have a hierarchical position but are able to facilitate collaboration because others trust their impartiality, judgment, and understanding of people. Figure 3.1 describes the three types of leaders as an integrated interactive team.

As Chapter 2 described, in the craft mode of production, physician leaders were master craftsman and were followed because of their knowledge of practice. This kind of professional hierarchy fits uncomfortably

**Figure 3.1   Integration of the Three Types
of Leaders into a Leadership Team**

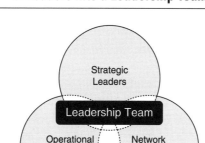

in many health care organizations today that are being pushed to become administered bureaucracies. Administrators are often pitted against physicians. But to become a learning organization, all professionals need to partner and fill leadership roles, as they do in some organizations we have studied, such as Intermountain and Jönköping in Sweden.

However, even some of the best organizations we've studied are not pure learning organizations. They combine craft, bureaucratic, and knowledge-based elements that fit their histories, cultures, and context. Intermountain Health Care (IHC) is a large integrated health system, with a health plan, dominant in its Utah and Idaho market. In comparison, Mayo Health Care (MHC) is a more acute care-focused academic health system, attracting patients from around the world, with a medical school and research arms supporting its "put the patient first" focus.

Leaders at IHC are partners, including nurses, administrators, MDs, and information technicians. Strategic, operational, and network leaders come from all disciplines. They work together on creating pathways and evidence-based medicine (EBM). This collaborative style of leadership, in which doctors interact in designing new procedures they will later practice, is crucial to earn physician buy-in. To gain agreement to follow new pathways, leaders need evidence to persuade physicians of their value. When multiple disciplines are involved, network leaders or operational leaders with networking qualities facilitate collaboration.

John E. Wennberg of Dartmouth and his colleagues have stated that "Intermountain is the best model in the country of how you can actually change health care for the better." He estimated that if health care were practiced nationally in the way it is provided at Intermountain, "the nation could reduce health care spending for acute and chronic illnesses by more than 40 percent."[2]

Mayo Health Care is also an exemplary model of a learning organization, but its unique history and culture differ from Intermountain. Administrator leaders at MHC are operational leaders or managers who serve physician leaders who earn their way up the hierarchy by proving their clinical and leadership competence. Mayo needs leaders with strategic intelligence to sustain its effectiveness, but because the learning culture has been established, exceptional visionary leaders are not essential. Mayo is still building on William Mayo's original vision. Both administrators and physicians practice Mayo's cultural values. MHC culture defines what leaders do and how they work together. Unlike at Intermountain, EBM and pathways are less central because MHC physicians see many complex, acute-care cases. Nonetheless, MHC has been working on pathways for less complicated cases. At MHC, physicians are salaried and work in teams from various clinical specialties determined by the needs of the patient. The MHC culture and style of leadership determines that physicians interact collaboratively in these treatment teams and learn from each other and the patient who is part of the team. Nurses at MHC may be operational or network leaders. The nurse who leads St. Francis hospital told Maccoby that nurses follow Mayo physicians not because they have superior hierarchical positions, but because they create mutual respect in the team by building trust and driving out fear.

What do these leaders, in any context, do to create change? In the knowledge and learning mode, strategic, operational, and network leaders work interactively to create shared purpose, practical values, and productive processes. Purpose, practical values, and processes are developed as a system, a vision essential to achieve the purpose. This vision is worked interactively through all levels and parts of the organization. In this way everyone comes to understand it.

Health care leaders will not create learning organizations if they act as ombudsmen for one group, such as physicians. They will gain support from all staff only if they are seen as advocates for the development of the whole organization in achieving its purpose. A study of "Organizational Factors Associated with High Performance in Quality and Safety in Academic Medical Centers" published in *Academic Medicine* found that the top leaders in the highest-performing academic hospitals had a hands-on, walk-around leadership style.[3] They often appeared inpatient care areas, and staff addressed them by first name. These leaders frequently told stories to illustrate the vision or pointed out organizational gaps that needed to be closed. They showed a willingness to learn from any staff member's concerns and ideas.

The most effective leaders of any organization model the organization's values. For example, top leaders and chairs in the best-performing academic medical centers described in the study in *Academic Medicine* accept personal responsibility for quality and safety results. These improvement processes are not programs they delegate and then sit back to wait for results. They are personally involved in developing and implementing the processes. They participate in forums for problem solving and idea generation. They assure that measurements of quality and safety are shared broadly with managers at all levels, as well as at the top and board levels of the organization. In these exemplary hospitals, there are on average 150 fewer deaths per year caused by mistakes than at the average academic hospital.

Leaders in a learning organization reach out to others outside their organization, in addition to seeking ideas and fresh thinking from their own front line. Operational leaders are encouraged by strategic leaders to make full use of new sources of learning. For example, IHC joined MHC, Dartmouth-Hitchcock, UCLA Health System, and Cleveland Clinic in a first-of-its-kind collaboration to achieve better patient outcomes and quality while reducing costs. These organizations will work together to create and implement best practices. One example of what they have accomplished is a better process for knee replacement.

How do leaders initiate change? CEOs may initiate the change process with discussions to define the purpose of the organization. For example, in the academic medical center study, the top-performing hospitals were led by a partnership of chairs (department heads) and executive leadership. The members of the leadership team were jointly responsible for program development and system improvements. Unlike piecemeal approaches to performance, the approach of these teams achieved a sustained critical examination and redesign of current processes.

Their collaborative approach proved an effective means to address chronic underperformance as a start to the change process.

When the organizational purpose is clear, leaders are ready to work out a systemic vision of how the organization will achieve that purpose. Chapter 6 will describe how an organizational vision aligns each element with the organization's purpose.

How a vision is developed and implemented can vary according to the unique elements of an organization. Many of the organizations in the academic medical center study determined strategic priorities and measures of outcomes centrally at the highest level, with board and operational level participation. Unit level leaders implemented the strategy. This is a tight-loose strategy for change, with priorities and outcome measures centrally determined, and implementation tactics developed differently in the various parts of the organization. There is no one best way. At IHC leaders encourage new ideas bubbling up from below. For example, the chief cardiologist assembled a leadership team of physicians, a chief nurse, and an administrator who studied treatment data prepared by the informatics department. This stimulated ideas for improvement in procedures that the team then brought to groups of cardiologists across the geographically dispersed system. Through these interactions everyone participated in creating the new procedures. This included questioning and discussion of all issues. In the process everyone became educated about the new procedures they helped create and was willing to practice them.

IHC has pioneered pathways that physicians have to follow unless they actively modify them. If they do so, the changes go back to the team that developed the pathway, and the team then decides whether or not the pathway should be modified.

Mayo implements its vision in part through its Value Creation System. To train implementers, Mayo has established an internal Quality Academy (IHC has a similar educational organization) which offers twenty-seven courses ranging from "overall strategy to more specific approaches/tools including lean, six sigma, change management, failure modes and effects analysis, project management, champions training, among others."[4]

The next chapters will describe more fully how to develop a leadership philosophy, the purpose and vision, and the kinds of knowledge and practices needed to lead change. These chapters will also provide the methods and tools leaders need to establish a learning organization.

SUMMARY

- Broad, effective leadership is needed to transform bureaucracies into learning organizations.
- Leadership is a relationship; management is a collection of functions.
- Three types of leaders—strategic, operational, network—need to work interactively.
- Good leaders make followers into collaborators by communicating a motivating philosophy and vision.

KEY TERMS

Leader, leadership

Management

Network leaders

Operational leaders

Strategic leaders

Transparency

Triple Aim

EXERCISES

1. Is your organization trying to become a learning organization? Why or why not?
2. Does your organization have strategic, operational, and network leadership? If not, what can you do to develop broad leadership for a learning organization?
3. What type of leader are you or do you aspire to be? What can you do to strengthen yourself as a leader?

ENDNOTES

1. Stephen J. Swenson, MD, James Dilling, BSIE, CMPE, C. Michael Harper Jr., MD, and John H. Noseworthy, MD, "The Mayo Clinic Value Creation System," *American Journal of Medical Quality* 27, no.1 (Jan/Feb 2012), 58–65.

2. J. E. Wennberg, J. S. Brownlee, E. Fisher, J. Skinner, and J. Weinstein, *An Agenda for Change: Improving Quality and Curbing Health Care Spending*, a Dartmouth Atlas White Paper (Lebanon, NH: Dartmouth Institute for Health Policy and Clinical Practice, 17 Dec. 2008).
3. Mark A. Keroack, MD, MPH, and others, "Organizational Factors Associated with High Performance in Quality and Safety in Academic Medical Centers," *Academic Medicine* 82, no. 12 (2007), 1178–1186.
4. Swenson et al., "The Mayo Clinic Value Creation System," 60.

4

DEVELOPING A LEADERSHIP PHILOSOPHY

To gain trust and support from the people you lead, they need to know what they can expect from you. How do you define the **purpose** of the organization you lead? What are the values you consider essential to achieve that purpose? What are the ethical and moral guidelines you use to make decisions? And how do you describe and measure goals and results? The most effective leaders of organizations provide answers to these questions and communicate them to all their collaborators.

Once you develop your answers to these questions, you will have articulated your **leadership philosophy**. A compelling leadership philosophy becomes a powerful tool for building an organizational culture with high levels of performance. It guides decision making, invites everyone in the organization to challenge practices that clash with the values that support the organization's purpose, and it provides guidelines for innovation at all levels.

Leaders will be trusted by collaborators who know and believe in the leaders' philosophy and competence—and when the collaborators are free to question whether the actions of the leaders are consistent with their philosophies. They will believe in a philosophy when they see a leader practicing it.

How to Develop a Philosophy

A comprehensive leadership philosophy includes at least four elements, based on the answers to these questions:

1. What is the purpose of this organization?
2. What ethical and **moral reasoning** determines the key decisions we make?
3. What **practical values** do we need to practice to achieve the purpose?
4. How do we define goals and results so they are consistent with our purpose and values?

Purpose

Purpose describes where and why a leader is leading an organization. A powerful statement of purpose will be meaningful to all stakeholders. Many organizations use *mission* to describe the organization's purpose. We find that "purpose" rather then "mission" implies a sustainable enterprise that connects more explicitly with clients and customers. Peter Drucker once stated that the purpose of business should not be just to make a profit just as the purpose of life is not to breathe. However, without either of these purposes, no other is possible. He believed that the main purpose of business is to gain and retain customers. Of course, even nonprofit health care organizations must gain enough revenue to pay salaries and to invest in continual improvement. But organizations won't succeed in gaining revenue if they do not attract patients and competent staff. In building his company, Henry Ford expressed a purpose of providing people with an affordable means of transportation. That was his way of gaining and retaining customers. Bill Gates described his purpose as improving the way people work. As long as Microsoft products do that, the company will gain and retain customers. William Mayo described his purpose as serving patients. At Intermountain Healthcare, Bill Nelson and Charles Sorenson described their purpose as not only serving patients at an affordable cost but also improving their quality of life.

Ethical and Moral Reasoning

Ethics has to do with following the rules, including the law, professional codes of conduct, religious commandments, and the principles that underlie these rules. Being ethical is essential to building trust. It also keeps someone out of serious trouble with law enforcement and regulatory agencies. Ethics should not only be part of every leadership philosophy, but also expected of everyone in the organization. However, the application of ethics depends on a leader's level of moral reasoning, which influences the leader's definition of the common good.

Levels of Moral Reasoning

Harvard psychologist Laurence Kohlberg[1] studied levels of moral reasoning and described the following three:

1. The lowest level defines the good as individual well-being, avoiding punishment or gaining rewards. This implies that a person conforms to ethical rules only when an authority is watching or might subsequently learn about an infraction. With this kind of morality, there is no common good. It's only looking out for number one.
2. The next level defines the good in terms of what people consider good for their family or organization as well as for themselves, without concern for the effect of their actions on those outside their circle. This definition can lead to a narrow view of the common good: we versus others. Or it can be a start of viewing self-interest in terms of the larger community that supports a group.
3. A broader definition of the common good is what benefits, or at least doesn't harm, all those who may be affected by one's actions. This might include employees, customers, owners, communities, unborn generations, and the natural environment.

At this third level of moral reasoning, leaders may be challenged to make tough decisions that don't benefit themselves or their organizations, but will benefit the larger common good. A decision like this requires moral courage. However, a decision that does not benefit an organization in the short term may do so for the longer term. A notable example was the 1982 decision by Johnson & Johnson's CEO to withdraw and destroy all Tylenol in stores because some capsules had been poisoned. This costly decision created trust in the company and its products.

Robert Wood Johnson crafted a company philosophy in 1943 that began "We believe our first responsibility is to the doctors, nurses and patients . . . who use our products." However, the company did not live up to this promise or the Tylenol example, when it waited nearly two years after receiving a warning from doctors before withdrawing a faulty hip implant from the market.[2]

The level of moral reasoning at which a leader and an organization operate can be inferred by the way that purpose, practical values, and definition of results are expressed. Examples of a high level of moral reasoning include

- **Google:** Sergey Brin and Larry Page, founders of Google, express the philosophy of "Do no harm." Their document "Ten Things We Know to Be True"[3] invites people to hold the organization accountable for acting in accordance with the ten things.
- **GE:** General Electric's slogan "We bring good things to life" has been used not just in marketing, but also to focus employees on the meaning of "good things" from the view of their customers, communities, and more recently, the environment.
- **The Mayo Clinic:** William Mayo built the Mayo Clinic on his philosophy that the patient comes first and Mayo doctors can challenge each other and authority according to whether their actions benefit patients.

By articulating a philosophy that includes a higher level of moral reasoning, you strengthen the focus on the patient and community and inspire your collaborators to think of the well-being not only of the patient and organization, but also of the supportive community.

Practical Values

Practical values express the beliefs and behaviors necessary to achieve the organization's purpose. These are the kind of values Bill Hewlett and Dave Packard of HP espoused and lived by. Their purpose was making products that were valuable to technical people because they helped them perform better. Their values included treating employees with respect, being loyal to them so they'd be loyal to HP, and contributing to their continual development. When there was a downturn of business, rather than laying anyone off, everyone took a cut in salary and time off; Hewlett's and Packard's view of the common good included customers, employees, the community, and investors. They also believed in hiring entrepreneurial people who would contribute to innovation.

Another value was collaboration; product developers who visited customers to learn about their needs worked as a team with manufacturing and marketing specialists. Their philosophy created trust and supported innovation from their technical staff. Over time, as HP grew, acquired companies, and brought in outsiders as CEOs, the HP philosophy (the "HP Way") was lost. Employees tell us that the company has suffered a loss of purpose and trust.

William Mayo's values included collaboration among different medical specialties and between doctors and nurses. Also essential was continual clinical research. Mayo travelled anywhere he could learn a new surgical method, and he returned to teach it at Rochester. Mayo created a patient-focused, collaborative culture of learning. In contrast to HP, Mayo leaders have affirmed their founder's philosophy and applied it to new clinics and projects.

Practical values to achieve quality, efficiency, and safety in a health care organization might include

- Respect for patients, their families, and staff
- Collaboration
- Learning from experience
- Sharing learning and using it to improve practice and processes
- Everyone participates in continual improvement
- Open communication
- Driving out fear so that people will speak freely
- Evidence based practice
- Judicious use of resources—only spending what a customer, owner, or citizen would consider necessary to achieve the organization's purpose.

Sometimes values will be in conflict. For example, there may not be time to gain collaboration to address an urgent problem. Or evidence-based practice may not fit a complex case. To be an effective leader, you need to be a **principled pragmatist**, someone who tests values in practice. Sometimes you will have to prioritize values or even modify how you define them. The key is always: how does this value support the organization's purpose?

Practical values may be called by different names: guiding principles, targeted behaviors, shared values, operational values. Regardless of what they are called, they need to be implemented to move the organization toward accomplishing its purpose.

We call these values "practical" because they are more than nice ideals. They are essential to achieving an organization's purpose. However, these values can also be rated according to whether or not they support the development of human qualities of collaboration, learning, individual responsibility, and critical thinking. Despite the nicely stated values of many organizations, the real values they practice reinforce conformity, rivalry, and groupthink.

Leaders need to know whether the values they espouse are being understood and practiced. Do people agree that these values are important to achieving the organization's purpose? And if so, how well are they being practiced? A way to discover this is by using a **gap survey**.

Gap Analysis

It can be valuable to conduct a survey using this format (see Table 4.1). Employees may have different views of the importance of these practical values and how well they are implemented. To deepen understanding of gaps between importance and performance, a leader should ask for the reasons for their ratings and examples that support these ratings.

When importance is higher than implementation, a leader should consider what can be done to communicate the importance or to create systems or reporting relationships that prioritize these practical values. Collaborators should be asked to suggest actions that would close the gaps. Then it is essential for leaders to follow through to strengthen the values that support the organization's purpose.

When implementation is higher than importance, leaders should consider whether the practical value may be seen as more important in

Table 4.1   Example of a Gap Survey

	How important is this value for achieving the organization's purpose?	How well are we practicing this value?
	1=Not Very Important; 5=Very Important	1=Not Practiced; 5=Practiced Very Well
Open Communication	1 2 3 4 5	1 2 3 4 5
Collaboration	1 2 3 4 5	1 2 3 4 5
Participation in Continuous Improvement	1 2 3 4 5	1 2 3 4 5
Shared Learning	1 2 3 4 5	1 2 3 4 5

some parts of the organization than in others, or whether resources are being focused on areas of lower importance and should be redirected.

Maccoby reports an example of a leader of an academic health center responding to a gap survey. The value of "service to the community" was considered important by some department chairs and unimportant by others. The leader asked representatives of each group to state the reasons for their scoring. Those who checked a score of 1 or 2 for importance said that the center was in financial trouble and couldn't afford pro bono service to the community. Those who checked 4 or 5 said that the community supported the center with transportation, security, and other services and freedom from taxes. If the center gave nothing back, it might lose support from the community. The leader agreed with this view and decided to increase services to the community. Those who were overruled went away satisfied that they had been heard, even though their views had not prevailed.

In Chapter 11, the use of gap surveys is described in more detail.

According to multinational and multi-organizational studies led by Berth Jönsson at Stockholm-based TNS SIFO, 70 percent of employees say that their employer has values that have been communicated to them—and 65 percent can name these values. However, only 47 of the 65 percent believe in and act on these values. This is only 31 percent of people who participated in the study—leaving 69 percent who do not believe in or act on the values that have been espoused.

Leaders in any organization that fits these statistics can affect great change by reaching two out of every three people with compelling practical values that they can believe in and act on.

Definition of Results

When a leadership philosophy is fully credible, the definition of results and the espoused values are fully consistent with the description of purpose.

Great health care organizations such as IHC and Mayo not only report financial results and quality and safety measures such as hospital mortality, adverse drug events, and surgical complications, but they also report measures of uncompensated benefits to the communities they serve. But these are all **trailing indicators**, describing past results. Future success depends on continued customer satisfaction and factors such as hiring, retraining, and developing talented people. The National Park Service defines results not only in terms of visitors and meeting budgets, but also in terms of environmental restoration and effective partnering including sharing technical information and expertise. By measuring trailing indicators, organizations can evaluate how well they have achieved their purpose. By measuring **leading indicators**, they keep track of the qualities essential for sustainable success.

IHC has defined results as

- Improved experience of care for the patient
- Reduced per capita cost for health care
- Application of learning from individual patients to improve the health of the community

IHC emphasizes that better quality of care invariably reduces costs because there is less rework—the same lesson that W. Edwards Deming taught the Japanese in 1950 and retaught America in the 1980s.

Results of projects as well as of the organization should include strengthening the system and its interactions. Results of decisions based on moral reasoning are best understood by the testimony of those involved. It's important to have quantitative goals that drive effective behavior. But inappropriate measurement can cause people to game rather than improve a system.

Using the Purpose to Define Results: Cherokee Nation Healthcare Services

Cherokee Nation Healthcare Services (CNHS) operates a network of eight health centers and one hospital which encompass fourteen counties of N.E. Oklahoma. During 2011 the leadership team of CNHS developed a purpose statement for the health care system:[4]

The Cherokee Nation Healthcare Services protects and promotes health and is the provider of choice through its workforce and in the delivery of a quality experience to those we serve while practicing good stewardship resulting in a happy and healthy Cherokee people.

The leadership team then used the purpose statement to identify the important measures for Cherokee Nation Healthcare Services. Table 4.2 describes the use of each statement in the purpose to identify the measures. Success on their "balanced scoreboard measures"[5] taken together help define results for Cherokee Nation Healthcare Services.

Table 4.2   Translation of the CNHS Purpose to System Level Measures

CNHS Purpose Statement	Balanced Scorecard Measures
"The Cherokee Nation Healthcare Services *protects and promotes health*	1. Immunization rates 2. Unadjusted raw mortality 3. Childhood obesity, ages 2–18 4. Morbidity
and is *the provider of choice*	5. Citizenry satisfaction rates 6. Percentage of third party 7. Active user population and visits 8. Percentage of patients empanelled 9. Average panel size per team/provider
through its *workforce*	10. Percentage of workforce Cherokee 11. Staff turnover rate 12. Productivity index 13. Incidence rate nonfatal occupational injuries and illnesses
and in the *delivery of a quality experience* to those we serve	14. Number of cancelled appointments 15. Adverse incidents 16. Third next available appointment 17. Equitable—inside fourteen county versus outside fourteen county
while *practicing good stewardship*	18. Health care costs per capita 19. Revenue per visit 20. Cost per visit
resulting in a *happy and healthy* Cherokee people."	21. Quality-of-life index 22. Disability associated life years

The Mayo Clinic Organization Philosophy

The Mayo Clinic has not organized its philosophy as we suggest here. However, its publications and the Annual Report of 2010 provide all the elements of a powerful organizational philosophy. Furthermore, Mayo leaders periodically review and affirm the organizational philosophy.

Rather then calling it purpose, Mayo describes a mission:

To inspire hope and contribute to health and well-being by providing the best care to every patient through integrated clinical practice, education and research.

The key concepts include integrated clinical practice and the clinical focus of education and research.

The needs of the patient come first. Mayo calls this their primary value. The practical values include the following:

- *Respect:* Treat everyone in our diverse community, including patients, their families and colleagues, with dignity.
- *Compassion:* Provide the best care, treating patients and family members with sensitivity and empathy.
- *Integrity:* Adhere to the highest standards of professionalism, ethics, and personal responsibility, worthy of the trust our patients place in us.
- *Healing:* Inspire hope and nurture the well-being of the whole person, respecting physical, emotional, and spiritual needs.
- *Teamwork:* Value the contributions of all, blending the skills of individual staff members in unsurpassed collaboration.
- *Excellence:* Deliver the best outcomes and highest quality service through the dedicated effort of every team member.
- *Innovation:* Infuse and energize the organization, enhancing the lives of those we serve through the creative ideas and unique talents of each employee.
- *Stewardship:* Sustain and reinvent in our mission and extended communities by wisely managing our human, natural, and material resources.

To practice these values, Mayo collaborates with numerous academic organizations throughout the world. Academic partnerships accelerate research, preventions and treatments for disease, as well as expand education and economic development opportunities in local communities. Mayo supports education and medical care for K–12 students in Minnesota schools and assists physicians in providing medical care to patients without insurance or the means to afford care.

Mayo describes measured results in terms of financials and the number of patients treated at its main locations in Minnesota, Arizona, and Florida. Also reported are the number of patients treated in the

Mayo Clinic Health System, a network of clinics and hospitals serving more then seventy areas in Iowa, Minnesota, and Wisconsin.

Every week Mayo randomly surveys patient satisfaction to learn about the patients' experience and to improve service. Quality is also measured in terms of mortality rates, surgical infections, safety, readmission rates, and compliance with evidence-based processes known to enhance care. Mayo also surveys employee attitudes to measure respect and teamwork.

Besides these, Mayo reports on the results of research and its efforts to improve the environment by increased use of renewable energy such as solar panels, recycling, and adding low-flow aerators to reduce water consumption.

Mayo provides results of charity care and its help for victims of floods in the United States and the earthquake in Haiti (2010 and 2011).

Leaders at Mayo can affirm the organizational philosophy and with gap surveys test whether or not they are being practiced. When we tested a group of Mayo leaders, we found little or no gaps between importance and performance. Mayo leaders walk the talk.

Some creative leaders have developed a leadership philosophy without calling it that. After Michael Choti at Johns Hopkins described how he leads his surgical team, Maccoby asked if he had a leadership philosophy. He said, "I haven't thought about it."

Maccoby said, "But you just told me that you encourage collegiality and first names on your team, because you want everyone to feel free to raise questions. You said you don't believe autocratic leadership works. However you affirm you are the leader and sometimes you have the responsibility to take charge and give directions. You explain carefully to the team and also to the patient and family what you believe needs to be done and the reasons why. After the operation you describe what you did and why you did it. You say your purpose is not only to perform successful surgery but also to lower the level of anxiety and create a relationship where patient, family and your collaborators feel free to ask questions and offer suggestions. That has elements of a philosophy: purpose, practical values, definition of good results. Probably, if you reflected on it, you could elaborate your philosophy."

"Yes," said Choti, "I think I could."

A final thought: whether or not we are aware of it, we all have personal philosophies, the purpose and values that give meaning to our lives. Your leadership philosophy will be convincing and authentic if it is consistent with your personal philosophy.

In Chapter 11, you'll be presented with a framework for describing your leadership philosophy.

SUMMARY

A comprehensive leadership philosophy includes at least four elements, based on the answers to these questions:

1. What is the purpose of this organization?
2. What ethical and moral reasoning determines the key decisions we make?
3. What practical values do we need to practice to achieve the purpose?
4. How do we define goals and results so they are consistent with our purpose and values?

As a leader it is important that your actions are congruent with your philosophy. People will then find it easier to understand your goals, strategies, and tactics as you work to achieve your vision. Your philosophy is a key communication tool.

KEY TERMS

Gap survey

Leadership philosophy

Leading indicators

Moral reasoning

Practical values

Principled pragmatist

Purpose

Trailing indicators

EXERCISES

1. What is the *purpose* of the health care organization where you are a leader? What should it be?

2. What are the *practical values* of the organization? What should they be?

3. Considering the purpose the organization should have, use the example in Table 4.2 (Cherokee Nation example) and develop some key measures for each statement in the organization's purpose. Do these measures reflect the results you desire today and in the future?

4. Begin developing your personal leadership philosophy by answering the following questions:

   • What is the purpose of the organization I lead? That organization may be a clinical department or administrative group that serves the clinical staff.
   • What ethical and moral reasoning determines the key decisions we make?
   • What practical values do we need to practice to achieve the purpose?
   • How do we define goals and results so they are consistent with our purpose and values?

ENDNOTES

1. Lawrence Kohlberg, "The Claim to Moral Adequacy of a Highest Stage of Moral Judgment," *The Journal of Philosophy* 70, no. 18 (1973), 630–646.

2. Barry Meier, "Doctors Who Don't Speak Out," *New York Times* (February 15, 2013).

3. Google, "Ten Things We Know to Be True," www.google.com/about/company/philosophy/ (accessed June 28, 2012).

4. Cherokee Nation Healthcare Services' (CNHS) purpose and associated measures were developed by the Jonathan Merrell and John Krueger for the CNHS Leadership Team. This was presented at the Southwest Quality Network Meeting April 25–26, 2012.

5. The Balanced Scorecard is a measurement device that attempts to present a group of measures that define the performance of an organization in a balanced fashion typically with measures for people, finances, operations, and community. Robert S. Kaplan and David P. Norton, "Putting the Balanced Scorecard to Work," *Harvard Business Review* (Sept.–Oct., 1993), 134–147.

PART 2

Strategic Intelligence and Profound Knowledge for Leading

5

LEADING WITH STRATEGIC INTELLIGENCE AND PROFOUND KNOWLEDGE

The leadership needed to make a complex health care organization a learning organization requires collaboration among leaders throughout the organization. This collaboration will be most productive when leaders share a common understanding of purpose and practical values, create a systemic vision of the organization, are able to design the processes and motivate people to implement the vision, and model learning from the organization's results. To achieve these aims, leaders at the top of the organization where strategy is crafted and a vision is designed are especially in need of the qualities of mind and heart that we term *strategic intelligence.*

Figure 5.1 has a dual meaning. The circles describe the qualities of heart and mind that interact with each other to strengthen the ability of leaders to continually adapt and learn as they shape and direct an organization. The arrows describe typical paths of leadership action that employs these qualities. However, while some leaders build a team to collaborate in designing an ideal future, others might design the vision before forming a team. As George E. P. Box noted, "All models are wrong; some are useful."[1] We offer this model as a useful introduction to a conceptual system made up of the following qualities:

- **Foresight:** Perception of the significance of events for your organization before they have occurred based on your subject

Figure 5.1   Strategic Intelligence, Leadership Philosophy, and Profound Knowledge

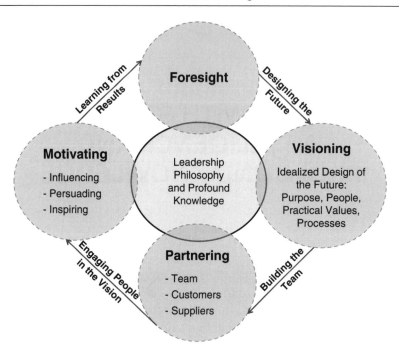

matter expertise, experience, research, scanning, and ability to sense dynamic trends.

- **Visioning:** Designing the future of the organization as a learning organization that can innovate and take account of the trends identified by foresight that indicate threats or opportunities for the organization. What is the idealized design of the organization as a social system for the future in terms of purpose, practical values, processes, and people?

- **Partnering:** Establishing productive relationships both internally and externally, based on mutual trust, common philosophy, and the sharing of risks and rewards.

- **Motivating:** Engaging people's intrinsic motivation by providing the *reasons* for people to help to realize the vision, defining motivating *relationships, responsibilities, rewards,* and *recognition* for contributions made to the organization.

Leaders should also be able to model learning from the organization's results and to make use of this learning in anticipating future trends. Let's consider briefly how each of these skills contributes to effectiveness in leading change of health care organizations.

Foresight

To design change, leaders should take account of the forces, described in Chapter 2, that are changing health care. These include the needs and attitudes of patients, new technology, public policy, and the costs and incentives resulting from these changes.

External Questions for the Organization:

1. What changes are taking place in the global health care community? How will these changes affect our delivery of care in the future?
2. What changes are taking place in the political and economic environments in which we operate? How will these changes affect the ways in which we operate (for example, the U.S. Affordable Care Act of 2010)?
3. What changes in technology could affect how we match the needs of our patients and families in the future? For example, how can technology help the patient with more effective self-care?
4. Will future needs of patients change the way we currently deliver care? Will our patients today be our patients tomorrow? Will our competitors' patients be our patients in the future? How can this cause a change in the way we operate in the future?
5. What will be the changes in the number or types of our competitors?
6. What will be the changes in our suppliers and their offerings?
7. What changes are we observing in the external environment that can be brought in and adapted to our organization to improve the quality and effectiveness of care delivered to our patients?

Internal Questions for the Organization:

1. What services will be required in the future?
2. What changes will this require of our organization?
3. What human resources will be required in the future? What skills will be required? What kinds of education and training will be required to stay current?

4. What changes will be required in the future in terms of capital and financial resources? Will we be expanding, decentralizing, or centralizing our health care operations?
5. What have we learned from the results and experiences that suggest future needs, opportunities, and challenges?

To Develop Foresight, Leaders Can Do the Following:

1. Scan the environment by communicating with experts and attending meetings where they present new ideas, reading about new technology, techniques, and legislation.
2. Develop scenarios about possible futures and work on contingency plans.
3. Join groups from other health care organizations that share findings. Serve on boards of exemplary organizations in health care and related fields.

Visioning as Designing the Idealized Organization

Visions are often wistful pictures of a more prestigious organization, such as "The number one provider for our patients." Or "The best care at the lowest cost." These are fine aims but they do not describe the idealized design of the future organization. In contrast, we define a *strategic vision* as a systemic blueprint of an ideal future which would achieve the organization's purpose more effectively and efficiently. Ackoff suggests three criteria for an idealized design of an organization.[2] They are

- *Technological feasibility:* The design should not incorporate any technology not currently known to be feasible. This does not preclude new uses of current technology. It is intended to prevent the design from becoming a work of science fiction.
- *Operational viability:* The organization should be designed to be capable of surviving in the current environment.
- *Learning and adaptation:* The organization should be designed so as to be able rapidly to learn from and adapt to its own successes and failures, and those of relevant others. It should also be capable of adapting to internal and external changes that affect its performance and of anticipating such changes (foresight) and taking appropriate action before such changes occur. This requires, among other things,

that the organization be susceptible to continual redesign by its internal and external stakeholders. The vision should be

- Developed by the leadership of an organization.
- Communicated, understood, and shared by the organization. People need to see how changes would benefit them and other stakeholders. This requires that all parts of the organization participate in the interpretation, development, and testing of changes that lead to effective implementation of the vision.
- Comprehensive and detailed. The vision should describe the organization as a system, aligning purpose with processes, roles and responsibilities, and practical values essential to achieving the purpose. To do this, leaders need a clear philosophy as described in Chapter 4 and the profound knowledge described in the following sections and chapters.
- Presented with a time frame of actions that will move the organization toward the ideal future. Chapter 11 presents exercises that can be used to chart the implementation process.

Partnering

Partnering is essential within and outside the organization. Leaders need partners with complementary skills and style. The leadership team needs all the qualities of strategic intelligence, and it's a rare leader who can do it all alone. For example, not everyone is good at the skill of foresight. The ability to develop productive partnering relationships is essential for creating effective leadership teams and building valuable relationships with provider, customer, and supplier organizations.

We have found there is a continuum in partnering with suppliers and organizational customers. A comprehensive partner-supplier program guides suppliers from being commodity suppliers through five levels of partnership arrangements (see Figure 5.2). Value-added suppliers have a framework agreement to provide a focused service, as FedEx has with the U.S. Postal Service (USPS) to handle airport-to-airport mail delivery, leaving the USPS with the local last-mile delivery. Alliance suppliers participate in joint development with the buyer, such as Intel with computer makers like HP. The learning consortium of Intermountain Health Care, Mayo, Cleveland Clinic, UCLA Medical Center, and others is an alliance to share innovations in treatment that improve quality

Figure 5.2   Partnering Continuum

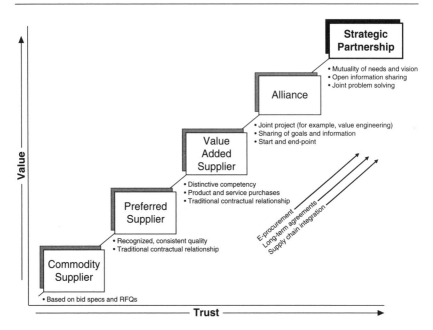

and lower cost. Strategic partners establish a common vision based on mutual needs and strategy, as Northwest Airlines and KLM had for fifteen years under the Wings Alliance before they merged in 2008. The Kaiser Hospital system and Permanente group of physicians is a strategic partnership. When he was CEO, David Lawrence forged a strategic partnership with the Kaiser Permanente unions. An early example of a partnership in health care is that of the Mayo brothers with the Sisters of St. Francis Hospital in 1885.

The Physician Group Incentive Program (PGIP) developed by Blue Cross Blue Shield of Michigan (BCBSM) is an exceptionally promising example of strategic partnering to increase quality, decrease per capita cost, and improve population health. BCBSM provides incentives for primary care providers, specialists, and facilities that create clinical integrated systems that best serve the community. The rewards for achieving the purpose go to the organization, not to individual physicians. The program includes shared information systems, processes of care, and continual learning among 40 physician led organizations (representing 92 smaller organizations) and almost 15,000 physicians. Organization size ranges from 25 to 1,600 doctors. These practices care for 5 million Michigan residents.[3]

David Share and Thomas Simmer of Blue Cross Blue Shield, who initiated the partnership, demonstrate the qualities of leadership described in this book. In an interview with Maccoby, Share emphasized: "system development and **transformation** are needed to achieve good results for patients and at a population level."

BCBSM promotes continual innovation and learning. According to an independent evaluation,

> With its intentional focus on harnessing physicians' intrinsic motivation, and recognizing the importance of fostering autonomy as an essential ingredient in inspiring full engagement in system change and outcome improvement efforts, BCBSM has encouraged a culture of collaboration among Physician Organizations, and between them and BCBSM. This is evidenced in the quarterly PGIP meetings, in a regional clinic process re-engineering collaborative, and in community-wide workgroups focused on challenges faced in common, such as registry implementation, data management and performance measurement. A unique effort known as the Care Management Resource Center emerged from collaborative discussions about the need for a central source of expertise and guidance for Physician Organizations engaged in implementing structured care management systems. PGIP serves as fertile ground for the development of such community-wide efforts which accelerate the pace of change, and elevate physicians' aspirations while providing practical support for realizing them.[4]

Companies that form true partnerships collaborate closely with partners to achieve not only lower total cost but also faster speed to market, more innovation, better quality, and safety for patients. The higher the level of partnering, the greater the level of trust required. Figure 5.3 provides some health care examples of these defined partnerships on the continuum.[5]

Figure 5.3   Partnering Continuum and Health Care Examples

Type of Relationship	Health Care Example
Commodity Supplier	Generic drugs, hospital supplies
Preferred Supplier	Doctors group
Value Added Supplier	Advisers for clinical and improvement knowledge
Alliance	Hospitals specialize and cooperate in a region
Strategic Partnership	Mayo Clinic and Sisters of St. Francis hospital

Motivating

We are all motivated by our internal needs and drives. We are motivated to eat, sleep, work, and to have fun. Work ties us to a real world that tells us whether or not our ideas make sense; it demands that we discipline our talents and master our impulses. To realize our potentials, we must focus them in a way that relates to others. We need to feel needed. Our sense of dignity and self-worth depends on being *recognized* by others through our work. Without work we deteriorate. We need to work; we need to make a contribution. The challenge for leaders is to engage people's internally driven motivation, the intrinsic motivation to work and contribute, to realize the vision.

Chapter 11 includes a diagnostic questionnaire that can be used to determine your strategic intelligence. There are also exercises to improve the qualities of strategic intelligence. Chapter 4 described the importance of a leadership philosophy in developing trust and clarity of purpose. A philosophy also strengthens strategic intelligence by directing foresight, describing the values that will be part of the vision, making sure that partners share purpose and values, and inspiring followers.

Profound Knowledge

To develop strategic intelligence, leaders also need to deepen their knowledge. Of course, this includes subject-matter knowledge of the health care business. Leaders also need to understand the interplay of theories of systems, variation, psychology, and knowledge. This understanding which W. E. Deming termed **profound knowledge** interacts with each element of strategic intelligence.

A leader of change doesn't have to be an expert in all of these fields. Deming advised us:

> One need not be eminent in any part of profound knowledge in order to understand it and to apply it. The various segments of the system of profound knowledge cannot be separated. They interact with each other. For example knowledge about psychology is incomplete without knowledge of variation.[6]

Leaders should partner with team members who complement their knowledge and talents. However, as Deming noted, a leader should

Figure 5.4   Lens of Profound Knowledge

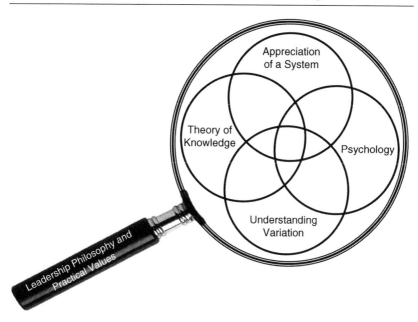

understand the basic theories in each area, how the different areas inter-relate, and why they are essential for success in leading change.

How leaders exercise foresight, partnering, visioning, and moti-vating will depend both on their leadership philosophy and profound knowledge. The following is a brief description of each area and how it interacts with strategic intelligence. In the chapters that follow, we will elaborate each area of profound knowledge.

Figure 5.4 shows the interrelationship among the elements of pro-found knowledge.

Understanding Systems

A learning organization is a **social system**. It can be defined as a collec-tion of interdependent processes and other elements with people work-ing interactively, guided by practical values, to accomplish the purpose of the system. None of the people, processes, or elements acting alone can do what the system does. Each component of a system should be evaluated only in terms of how well it furthers the system's purpose.

The parts of a **mechanical system**, like an automobile, can be designed to work together to further the system's purpose: transportation. The parts of **organic systems**, like the human body, are genetically designed to further the purpose of living. An organization is a social system, a collection of interdependent processes and other elements with people working interactively, guided by practical values, to accomplish the purpose of the system. Some parts can be designed, such as technology, roles, and processes, and other parts must be led, so that people who come to work with their own purposes share a common purpose.

We have stated in Chapter 4 that leaders should communicate a philosophy that clarifies

- *Purpose:* The definition of the purpose of the organization that defines the system's aim.
- *Practical values:* Behavior essential to achieving that purpose, including ethical and moral reasoning.
- *Results:* Definition of results for the system.

This leadership philosophy helps to integrate an organizational system. The leadership team also has the task of acquiring the technology and designing the roles and work processes that further the system's purpose.

Keep in mind that each element of any system should be evaluated not in isolation, but in terms of how well it interacts with other components in the system and furthers the system's purpose. Russell Ackoff, who developed our understanding of systems, used to give the example of finding the best auto parts from different models of cars. He pointed out that if you put together the best engine from one car with the best braking system, clutch, drive train, and so forth, from other cars, you'd end up with a pile of parts that wouldn't fit together to accomplish the purpose of transportation. Yet many organizations are designed like this, boasting of the best production facility, marketing and engineering departments, and so on, without evaluating how these departments interact and contribute as a system to the organization's purpose. So it may be with health care organizations that advertise different specialties without integrating them in a system with the aims of improving patient health, improving community health, and reducing the per capita cost of health care. The success of a learning organization will depend on the integration of its elements, not the performance of individual parts. This understanding will aid in making decisions about both the design of the system and improvements to it. Furthermore, systems usually operate within a larger system to which they must adapt. Cars are designed differently to adapt to superhighways or mountain roads, and to the availability and price of gasoline. Health care organizations must adapt to environmental factors, such as urban versus rural settings; national policy differences; cultural differences; and different demographics, such as the ages of patients.

A challenge for leaders of health care organizations is to

1. Partner with their teams to design a learning organization, a system that can deliver care while continually increasing quality and lowering costs.
2. Design a structure of roles and processes that makes it easy for people who come to work with their own purposes to collaborate to create the learning organization.

More about systems will be described in Chapter 6.

Understanding Variation

In any organizational system, leaders are faced with variation and the need to make decisions based on how variation is interpreted and understood. Have our infection rates been reduced? Are the efforts we have been making with diabetes patients over the past few months showing improvement in the hemoglobin A1C index? Do the medication errors in our hospital indicate a dangerous trend? Was the improved performance this week the result of changes we made, or was it just luck? How do we account for changes in the readmission rate at our hospital? To make effective improvements, it is essential to understand the theory of variation.

Walter Shewhart, a pioneer in understanding variation, observed that when data is plotted over time, the patterns may be either predictable or unpredictable. Based on these observations, Shewhart distinguished between *common causes* and *special causes* of variation over time in systems.

Common causes: those causes inherent in the process over time that affect everyone working in the process, and that affect all outcomes of the process.

Special causes: those causes *not* part of the process all the time or that do not affect everyone, but arise because of specific circumstances.

A process that has only common causes affecting the outcomes is called a *stable process*, or one that is in a state of *statistical control.* In a stable process, the causal system of variation remains essentially constant over time. This does not mean that there is no variation in the outcomes of the process, nor that the variation is small, or that outcomes meet requirements. It only implies that the variation is *predictable* within statistically established limits. If the system is not meeting requirements or the outcomes are not desirable, this indicates that a fundamental change to the system is needed for improvement.

A process whose outcomes are affected by both common and special causes of variation is called an *unstable process.* An unstable process is not necessarily one with large variation. Rather, the magnitude of variation from one period to the next is unpredictable. If special causes can be identified and removed, the process becomes stable, and performance becomes predictable. In practical terms this implies that improvement can occur by identifying the special causes and taking appropriate action. Once a change is made, continuing to plot data over time and observe the patterns helps to determine whether the change is an improvement and may alert you to new sources of variation, some of which may occur because of the changes you have made. In Chapter 7, we will describe how you can make use of your knowledge of variation.

Understanding Psychology

Both partnering and motivating require understanding yourself and the people you work with and lead. Understanding people means understanding what motivates them and how they interact with each other. This understanding helps leaders to predict how people will respond to their initiatives, why they embrace or resist change, and what it takes to engage them in collaboration.

We all have the tendency to view our own behavior as a rational response to a situation, while viewing the behavior of others as expressing their personalities. However, we all have values and motives that interact with our interpretation of a situation. In Chapter 8, we'll describe the elements of personality, including

- What we are uniquely born with—our *talents* and *temperament*
- How we are like others who have grown up in the same culture—our *social character*
- How we are like some people within our culture—our *motivational type*
- How are we like all people—our *drives*
- How we are like no one else—our *identity* and *philosophies*

What motivates us at work? And how can leaders effect this motivation, especially when leading change?

The strongest and most sustainable motivation engages our *intrinsic* values and skills. We are intrinsically motivated to work at tasks that are meaningful and challenging with others who are respectful and supportive, who make us hopeful about our future, and who recognize our achievements. In contrast, pay is an *extrinsic* motivator. It may cause a person to change behavior, for example, motivating a doctor to see more patients. But it won't motivate a professional to do a better job or to follow a leader enthusiastically. The lack of fair pay causes resentment and may be demotivating. And the problem with bonuses is they create the expectation of continued rewards. Even nonmonetary rewards can be demotivating if they are based on an authority's evaluation that honors one person over another, especially if the authority plays favorites.

Understanding Theory of Knowledge

A vision, or for that matter any change, is a prediction—a prediction that if the change is made, improvement will result. The more knowledge leaders have about how the particular system functions or could function, the better their predictions and the greater the likelihood that the changes they are leading will result in improvement. Comparing predictions to results is a key source of learning for leaders and leadership teams.

Predictions are based on theories. Any theory we have represents our current knowledge about how some aspect of the system works or what we believe will happen in the future (foresight). When is our theory valid enough to begin testing our ideas for change? When leaders make theories (or hypotheses) explicit, this will guide people in an organization as they carry out targeted improvement efforts to accomplish the vision, which is a prediction about the ideal future of the organization.

When leaders state their theories or assumptions, this also helps people design tests to validate these theories and make improvements from the results of these tests.

How do we learn? The journey is not necessarily linear. Learning may be advanced by iteration. An initial hypothesis leads by a process of deduction to predictions of necessary consequences that may then be compared with data. When consequences and data fail to agree, the discrepancy can lead, by induction, to modification of the hypothesis. A second cycle in the iteration is thus initiated. The consequences of the modified hypothesis are worked out and again compared with data. That in turn can lead to further modification and knowledge gain.

Leaders can also learn by testing their values in practice. Chapter 4 states that a leadership philosophy includes the organization's purpose and the practical values essential to achieving that purpose. These values will be understood only in terms of the behavior they shape. If they do not produce behavior that supports the organizational purpose, they must be better taught, enforced, or modified. In this sense, the values of a leadership philosophy are similar to a normative theory. They predict the behavior essential to achieve the organization's purpose. Chapter 9 expands on the challenge of developing knowledge in a learning organization.

Employing Strategic Intelligence and Profound Knowledge

Strategic intelligence, profound knowledge, and a meaningful leadership philosophy are the qualities and conceptual tools that equip a leader of change. However, they do not provide formulas for action. Decisions require good judgment and courage. Sometimes, information is inadequate. Leaders may not be certain about an investment. They may have doubts about selecting someone as a leader. As they develop strategic intelligence and profound knowledge, their judgment will be strengthened. But making decisions, despite reasonable doubt, requires courage, the quality that guarantees all the others.

In the chapters that follow, we expand on these qualities and what it takes to develop them.

SUMMARY

- The four parts of strategic intelligence have been introduced:

  - Foresight: perception of the significance of events for your organization before they have occurred based on your subject matter expertise, experience, research, scanning, and ability to sense dynamic trends.
  - Visioning: use of the idea of idealized design; designing the ideal system for the future.
  - Partnering: both internally and externally to the organization.
  - Motivating: use of the Five Rs of motivation, reasons, responsibilities, relationships, rewards, and recognition.

- The four parts of profound knowledge for leaders have been overviewed. A chapter on each component will be covered later in the book:

  - Theories of systems: understanding the organization viewed as a system as opposed to a focus on the organizational hierarchy.
  - Understanding variation: appreciation of the difference between *special* and *common* cause variation when making decisions about data and information.
  - Understanding psychology: the human side of change.
  - Theory of knowledge: how we learn and perceive the world.

KEY TERMS

Foresight

Mechanical system

Motivating

Organic system

Partnering

Profound knowledge

Social system

Visioning

EXERCISES

1. Consider the questions under foresight for both the internal and external view of the organization presented in this chapter.
2. Russell Ackoff presented a provocative question: If you could do anything you wanted in your organization without constraints, how would you design your organization? Ackoff then adds: "If you don't know what to do if you could do anything you want, how could you possibly know what to do if you could not do anything you want." Consider this provocation for your organization.

ENDNOTES

1. George E. P. Box and Norman R. Draper, *Empirical Model-Building and Response Surfaces* (New York: Wiley, 1987), 424.
2. The concept of idealized design has been taken from the work of Russell Ackoff; more can be read in the book, *Idealized Design: How to Dissolve Tomorrow's Crisis . . . Today*, by Russell L. Ackoff, Jason Magidson, and Herbert J. Addison (Upper Saddle River, NJ: Wharton School Publishing, 2006).
3. David A. Share and others, "How a Regional Collaborative of Hospitals and Physicians in Michigan Cut Costs and Improved the Quality of Care," *Health Affairs* 30, no. 4 (April 2011), 636–645.
4. David Share, MD, MPH, Blue Cross Blue Shield of Michigan, "From Partisanship to Partnership: The Payor-Provider Partnership Path to Practice Transformation," Testimony Submitted to the House Ways and Means Committee, Health Subcommittee, February 2012.
5. David Jacoby, *Guide to Supply Chain Management* (New York: Bloomberg Press, 2009), 167; Michael Maccoby, "Learning to Partner and Partnering to Learn," *Research Technology Management* 40, no. 3 (May-June, 1997), 55–57.
6. W. Edward Deming, "A System of Profound Knowledge," Ch. 11 in *The Economic Impact of Knowledge,* ed. Dale Neef, G. Anthony Siesfeld, and Jacquelyn Cefola (Woburn, MA: Butterworth-Heinemann, 1998).

6

CHANGING HEALTH CARE SYSTEMS WITH SYSTEMS THINKING

Daphne Tan, MD and CEO of a hospital group in Asia, had just finished reading a book by Russell Ackoff on systems thinking. She was intrigued by the prospect of applying systems thinking to health care. She decided to call in Andrew Chow, MD, who had just finished his third project as an improvement professional. "Dr. Chow, what do you know about systems thinking?" Daphne asked. Dr. Chow answered, "Dr. Tan, during one of our workshops we learned about Dr. W. Edwards Deming and his idea of the organization viewed as a system as opposed to the organization viewed on an organizational chart. It has really changed the way I think." Dr. Tan asked, "Dr. Chow, do you think you could prepare a short presentation for our leadership team on Deming's idea and systems thinking?" Dr. Chow welcomed the opportunity. "When would you like this presentation to happen?" Dr. Chow asked. Dr. Tan said, "Would our next meeting of the staff be too soon?" Dr. Chow replied, "Not at all. I am looking forward to it."

Health care organizations are extremely complex. A complex bureaucracy can't be transformed into a learning organization just by improving practices in each department. In a learning organization, each department's processes interact with others to achieve the organization's purpose of improving patient health and quality of service while reducing per capita costs. Multiple processes from various departments routinely interact in diagnosis and treatment. Implementing best practices to avoid suboptimization requires systems thinking. In a learning organization, "hard" organizational factors like defined roles, processes, and measurements are supported by "soft" factors like leadership style and shared values.

Designing an idealized vision of the organization and describing how both hard and soft factors interact to achieve the purpose of a health care organization requires viewing the health care organization as a social system. In Chapter 5, we described a social system as a collection of interdependent processes and other elements with people working interactively; guided by practical values, to accomplish the purpose of the system. We also contrasted three types of systems: mechanical, organic, and social.

> Dr. Tan introduced Dr. Chow to the leadership team. Dr. Chow had worked with many of the leaders before. Dr. Tan gave a brief overview of systems thinking and then gave Dr. Chow the floor. During the presentation the VP of purchasing and administration, Wendy Goh Chin, asked, "Dr. Chow, recently I read an article where people believe it is useful to view the organization as a complex adaptive system. Can you explain how this relates?" Dr. Chow answered, "Great question. This idea of the **complex adaptive systems** or CAS is often used as a metaphor for how organizations work as a system. This is the type that Russell Ackoff termed the *animated* or *organic* system. It is useful as a metaphor because it helps people think about self-organizing and collaboration. However, we are talking about the organization as a social system. Let me explain the important differences."

Some leaders have tried to construct organizations as mechanical systems, bureaucracies where employees are programmed to perform repetitive work. But employees treated as machine parts tend to turn off. They are not motivated to cooperate or to use their brains to improve the system. Nor is it useful to think of a health care organization as a self-organizing organic system, like ants or bees organizing themselves to find food. The purpose and behavior of an organic system are determined genetically; a health care organization requires that leaders determine the system's purpose and create the collaboration necessary to achieve it, in effect creating a social system where the people who work in the system and the system itself have purposes. In other words, each is making choices and leadership is required to ensure that there is a common purpose and that all parts of the system are aligned to achieve that purpose.

A learning organization is a social system unlike a mechanical or organic system; the people in a social system—doctors, nurses, technicians, and administrators—may all bring different values and purposes to the organization. Without leadership there would be no common purpose or values. Figure 6.1 describes the transformation from viewing the organization as an organization of people reporting to each other to viewing it as a system where the patient (customer) is the focus of the system.

To create a social system as a collaborative learning organization, it is useful to employ the following Four Ps that follow from the definition of a social system:

- *Purpose:* What is the purpose of our organization? Who are we serving? What value do we add for them?
- *Processes:* How are our work processes linked to make the system achieve its purpose effectively and efficiently? What do we measure? Processes produce products and services and these are outputs of the system. One might consider products and services as the fifth P.
- *People:* What are the roles and responsibilities we need to fill and what kinds of people do we need to fill them? What are the skills they need to have? How should they interact? What kinds of personality traits are we looking for? What kinds of relationships do we need to manage?
- *Practical values:* What are our values and how do they support the system's purpose?

Figure 6.1 Transforming from an Organizational Focus to a Health Care System Focus

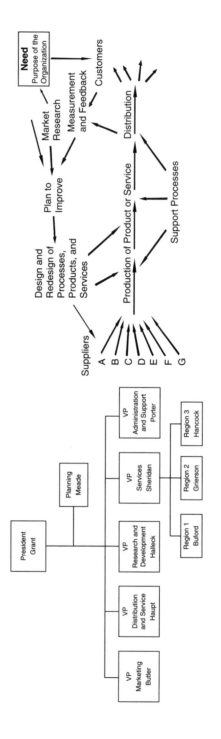

Figure 6.2   An Organization Viewed as a System

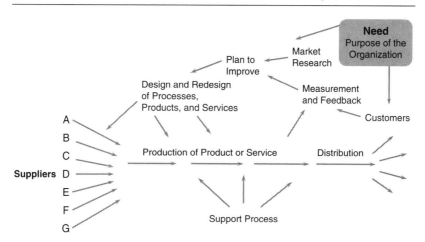

Source: Gerald J. Langley, Ronald D. Moen, Kevin M. Nolan, Thomas W. Nolan, Clifford L. Norman, and Lloyd P. Provost, *The Improvement Guide: A Practical Approach to Enhancing Organizational Performance*, 2nd ed. (San Francisco: Jossey-Bass, 2009), p. 313.

W. Edwards Deming viewed the processes of an organization as a system (see Figure 6.2.). He saw the role of management as designing and continually improving the system, much like a conductor leading an orchestra.

Deming described the *purpose* of the organization as meeting needs in society. In his system, there is a continual effort to match products and services to these needs and to improve products and *processes* for the benefit of customers and clients. Leaders are responsible for anticipating the future needs of customers and ensuring that the organization aligns to this future; Deming called this alignment, "creating constancy of purpose."[1] To help ensure constancy of purpose for the future, leaders must communicate the *practical values* of the organization to help *people* achieve shared meaning. A typical organization chart shows the reporting lines for departments, staff groups, and individuals. That view presents the organization as a bureaucracy based on command and control (see Figure 6.3).

That chart describes formal responsibilities, but not the production system of a service organization, including how services are developed and delivered and who interacts with customers and suppliers. Figure 6.4 shows the names on the organization chart (from Figure 6.3) placed on the flow diagram of production as a system (Figure 6.2). Individuals can now see how their jobs in specific work processes support the purpose of the system.

Figure 6.3   Organization Chart for a Service Organization

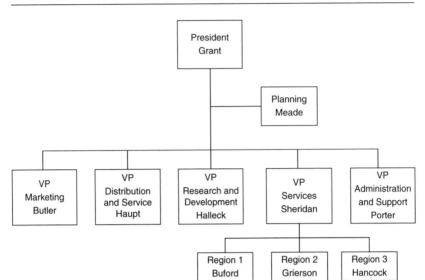

Figure 6.4   Systems View of a Service Organization

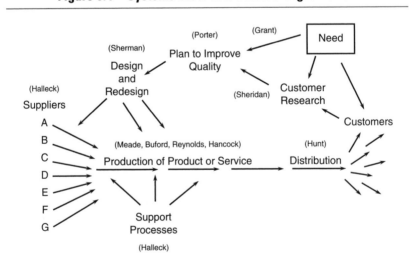

Dr. Chow explained, "Mental models influence how people act. When we have an organizational chart as a mental model, we tend to treat the boss as the customer and work in silos. When we look at the organization as an interdependent system, we clearly see which processes touch our internal customers, patients, and their caretakers." Many of the leaders in the room saw the implications and began to question this notion. Dr. Rachel Dali, medical director, then asked, "What is the impact on our roles and authority?" Dr. Chow thanked Dr. Dali for her question and explained, "This view of how the system works puts the focus on taking care of patients first and foremost. All of us have important roles to make certain that the purpose of the health care system is achieved. Furthermore, it is part of our job as leaders to help people understand the importance of their roles and relationships within the system to enable collaboration between people and other processes or departments. All of us understand the danger of handoffs in our system. This systems view helps to safeguard patient safety and satisfaction." Rachel Dali immediately saw the benefit and responded, "So, Dr. Chow, this model actually puts everyone to work on the purpose and our job as leaders is to make sure we have properly aligned people to provide the best care for our patients." Dr. Chow replied, "Dr. Dali, I think that is a good summary. The key is to understand that all work is a process and those processes are interconnected. We need everyone to be focused and learning together to reduce the potential for harm and increase our ability to deliver the best possible care to our patients. Let's discuss some more ideas around the idea of systems thinking."

Systems thinking means viewing the learning organization as adaptive to the needs of patients, providers, and all employees and comprised of interdependent people, equipment, products, and processes, all working toward a common purpose. The leaders of the organization are responsible for orchestrating the components of the system to achieve its purpose and to ensure that learning is taking place to establish constancy of purpose.

Systems thinking is essential when leaders develop, test, and implement changes to a system. Making fundamental changes to a small part of a system can lead to suboptimization and unintended consequences for the larger system when the impacts of these changes are not considered and understood. As stewards of the system, leaders are responsible for thinking and learning about the impact of proposed changes on the system, its patients, families, and other stakeholders today and in the future.

Interdependence

Interdependence means that components of a system do not work independently. This idea can be best understood by looking at two specific examples.

1. Each member of a four-person bowling team improves his or her average by ten pins. What is the impact on the team's score?
2. Each of four department managers in a health care organization carries out changes that cut monthly costs by $10,000 in his or her department. What is the monthly savings to the organization?

One is tempted to apply the same arithmetic to each example (for example, the bowling team increased its total score by forty pins and the organization obtains a $40,000 monthly savings in costs). In the bowling example, there is very little interdependence in the team. The output of each team member is additive to the result of the team.

In the second example, the assumption of summing up each of the department's contributions to cost reduction may not hold. The departments (for example, administration, purchasing, operating room, and the emergency department) may have many interactions that make them interdependent. The amount of cost savings calculated in one department may have a smaller or larger effect when costs are measured for the whole organization. For example, a savings by the purchasing department on purchased supplies may result in significantly increased setup and rework costs in the operating room. The net result for the organization may be an increase in total cost, not a savings.

The second step in developing a systems view of an organization is to recognize that the organization is composed of individuals, groups, departments, and processes, whose performances all affect and are dependent on other individuals, groups, and departments. If the system is highly interdependent, leadership is necessary to manage the interactions of the system. Understanding these interactions and the corresponding social relationships is necessary to ensure that the purpose of the system is achieved while creating an environment where intrinsic motivation can flourish.

> During his presentation Dr. Chow wanted to make sure that everyone appreciated the idea of work as a process. In many work situations, he often heard people use the word "process," but when it really came to understanding work as a process there was a skill to be developed. Dr. Chow explained, "Several times during this presentation we have discussed the concept of work as a process. Let's spend some time on defining what we mean by the word process."

What Do We Mean by Process?

All work can be described as a process. A *process* can be defined as a set of causes and conditions that repeatedly come together in a sequence of steps to transform inputs into outcomes. Figure 6.5 describes the concept of a process.

Processes can be described by a flow diagram that usually has a beginning and end with activities and decisions over time. Systems can be composed of subsystems with processes nested within each subsystem. In developing a linkage diagram, we need to focus on the key processes in an organization.

Figure 6.5   Concept of a Process

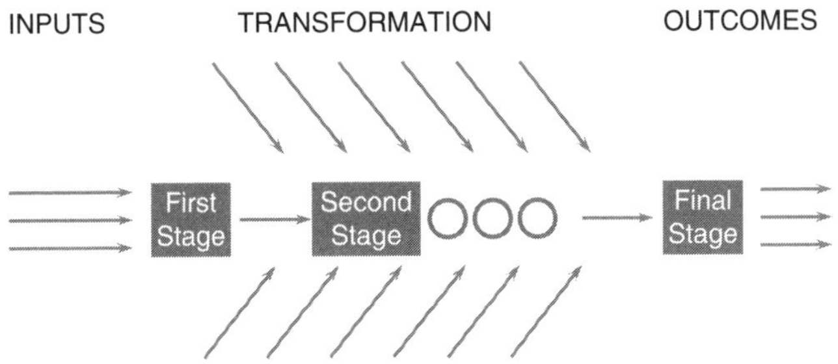

Figure 6.6   Concept of a Key Process and Level of Detail in Nested Systems

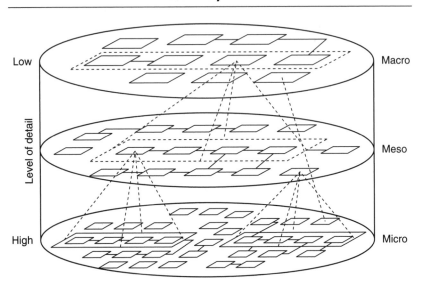

Source: Gerald J. Langley, Ronald D. Moen, Kevin M. Nolan, Thomas W. Nolan, Clifford L. Norman, and Lloyd P. Provost, *The Improvement Guide: A Practical Approach to Enhancing Organizational Performance,* 2nd ed. (San Francisco: Jossey-Bass, 2009).

Figure 6.6 describes the concept of a **key process** as viewed at different levels of detail with nested systems. The top of the diagram (low level of detail or macro view) represents the view of the top managers of the organization: the linkage of processes as developed for the entire organization. This linkage could contain key processes from the other three levels.

Key processes are those essential for accomplishing the aim of a system. They collectively include the work of more than 90 percent of those working in that system. Managers will usually have direct, detailed knowledge of these processes and the reason why they are essential for achieving the system's purpose.

An example of a key process comes from a system of hospice care. Joint planning with the family and providers produces a care plan for a specific patient including diet, nutrition, special issues, meds, and end-of-life issues. The care plan determines downstream processes where errors can occur from handoffs.

Leaders of the system should be aware of processes like this and understand their leverage in the system. A problem we've observed is that some executives do not update their knowledge of key processes that they understood years before when they were directly involved in managing them. Decisions based on outmoded knowledge of key processes cause confusions and worse.

Note that on the chart in Figure 6.6, one of the key processes with a high level of detail is also a key process when viewed at a low level of detail. This is a key process in its own right and is listed as such in the overall linkage. Also, three key processes in the midlevel of detail are shown as only one key process in the linkage with the lower level of detail.

> As Dr. Chow continued his presentation on systems thinking, he next focused on complexity. "We all appreciate how complex health care delivery systems can be. When we make changes it is very important that we understand that there are two kinds of complexity to consider. Using a systems view can help us understand and predict the impact of our changes on important outcomes for our patients and the results we expect."

Two Kinds of Complexity

Figure 6.7 describes an effort made by a VP in an organization to change a process at the third level of the nested systems (see Figure 6.6). From this figure we can discuss two basic types of complexity in a system: **detailed complexity** and **dynamic complexity**. If we have an understanding of the nested systems, we can deal with the effects of detailed and dynamic complexity. However, if we drill down from only the knowledge of the organizational chart, we could be in trouble with a change in detail. Many conventional analysis methods try to deal with detailed complexity through study of the many variables in a system and understanding cause and effect relationships. The process to be changed is represented by the standard flow diagram shapes of rectangles, diamonds for decisions, and so on. It is great that a change is being made (detailed complexity). However, while making this change, it may be very important to understand the impact of this change throughout the system (dynamic complexity).

In industry, such a change might result in unintended consequences of increased costs or unhappy customers. In health care, this change

Figure 6.7   Nested Systems and Change at the Detail Level

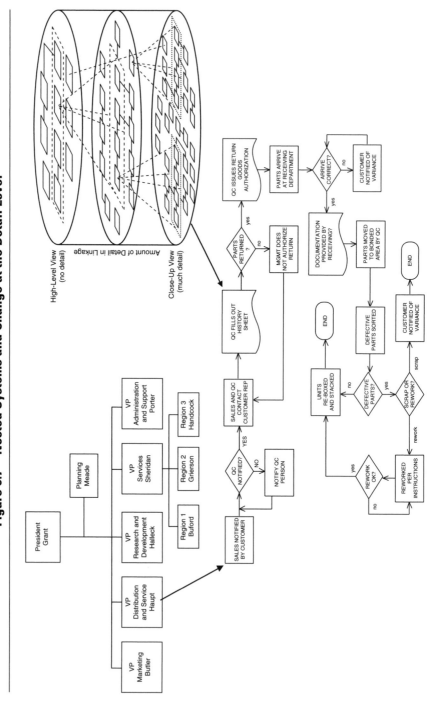

could result in a patient safety incident or other harm in addition to economic consequences. A key use of the systems view is to help ensure that changes are properly integrated to improve systems integrity. In Figure 6.7 we can take immediate action at this third level in the system and we may see an immediate benefit in the process depicted by the flow diagram (detailed complexity). Many changes we make in a system have a very different effect in the short run and long run; this is called dynamic complexity or temporal complexity. With dynamic complexity, delayed effects are a common expectation and cause and effect is not necessarily close in time or space.

From a health care perspective we could think of a health care system in a major city or region of a country that might have three hospitals and thirty-five primary care clinics. This would be at the macro level. The meso level might show a systems design for a single hospital. The micro level might describe the emergency department as a system.

Dr. Tan interjected a statement at this point in the discussion relative to detail and dynamic complexity and the nested levels in a system. "Dr. Chow, it is very clear to me that we need to have some view of the system to really understand the impact of detailed changes to our health care system in order to proactively make certain that we don't suffer unintended consequences. We tend to assume changes will result in improvements. But I am beginning to see that without considering the dynamic complexity, we can easily overlook the system impact of that change. In other words, a change that helps my area may actually hurt the system somewhere else." Dr. Chow responded, "Dr. Tan, that is an excellent point. This leads to our next discussion on how to get a shared understanding of the system. This task begins with understanding the three types of work processes that make up our system."

Classifications of Processes

When constructing a **linkage of processes**, it may be useful to think about different groupings of processes. Figure 6.8 shows the production

Figure 6.8   Three Types of Processes

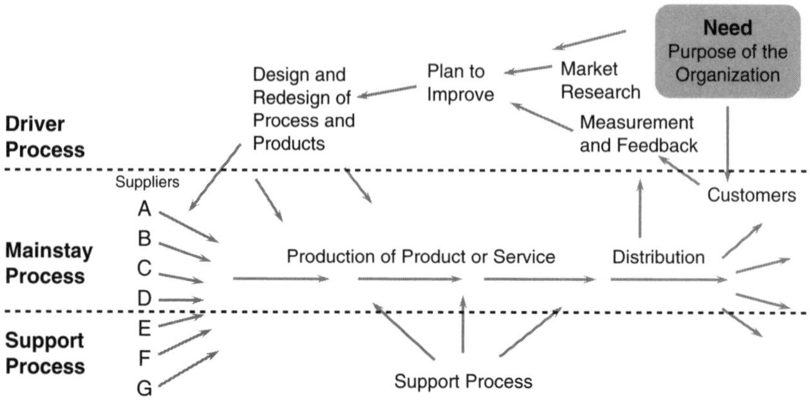

Source: Quality as a Business Strategy (Austin, TX: API-Austin, 1998). Available online from http://www.pipproducts.com/books.html.

viewed as a system diagram with the location of the three types of processes identified.

The first group, "mainstay" processes, represents the primary business of the organization. The **mainstay processes** are identified in the purpose statement because they are the processes that directly support the purpose of the organization. The word "mainstay" is a nautical word referring to the support rope that connects the mainmast of a sailing ship to the foremast. The mainstay of the business denotes what we do in the system that directly adds value for the external customers of the system; we could think of the mainstay as the delivery system with which patients and families directly interact. Describing the processes that form the mainstay of the health care organization is usually a good first step in building a linkage of processes. Chapter 10 contains several examples of systems maps for health care organizations and some discussion that can help you develop a systems view for your organization. Chapter 11 describes the steps for developing a systems view for your organization.

In his book, *The Competitive Advantage of Nations*, Michael Porter discusses how "competitive advantage grows out of the way firms organize and perform discrete activities."[2] He groups the various activities into categories that form a "value chain." Porter defines an organization's value chain as an interdependent system or network of activities connected by linkages. These linkages also connect the organization to suppliers and customers outside the system. Porter states that gaining competitive advantage requires that a firm's value chain is managed as a system rather than a collection of separate parts. The processes that form Porter's value chain are the mainstay processes.

The Institute of Medicine's (IOM) *Crossing the Quality Chasm* report proposes ten new simple rules as a framework for the enhancement of the effectiveness of delivery systems (mainstay) in health care.[3] Each rule is presented in juxtaposition to the prevailing, and less helpful, current design rule. As you review Table 6.1, note that improved practice assumes the shift in care we discussed earlier in Chapter 2 from the craft-independent system to learning organization. By understanding the underlying system, you will be better able to ensure that processes are defined with simple rules for improved practice built into the process and roles of people performing these processes. The case studies in Chapter 10 describe several examples of leaders defining systems and integrating the roles of people into their systems. Without this work, changes may not be sustainable.

In summary, mainstay processes are defined as follows: those processes that directly relate to the purpose of the organization and add value to the external customers of the organization.

Besides the mainstay or delivery processes, it is useful to identify two other types of processes in an organization:

- **Driver processes:** those processes that drive the mainstay of the organization. These processes are usually associated with the needs the organization intends to fulfill and are located in the top part of the production viewed as a system model (see Figure 6.8). Examples of driver processes are customer feedback, planning, research, development, and budgeting. These processes get the organization ready to match the need when performing its mainstay processes.
- **Support processes:** those processes that are necessary to support the mainstay processes. Examples include accounting, maintenance, hiring, traveling, and handling communications.

Table 6.1   Institute of Medicine's Ten Simple Rules for Delivery Systems

Current Practice	Improved Practice
1. Care is based primarily on visits.	1. Care is based on continuous healing relationships.
2. Professional autonomy drives variability.	2. Care is customized according to patients' needs and values.
3. Professionals control care.	3. The patient is the source of control.
4. Information is a record.	4. Knowledge is shared freely.
5. Decision making is based on training and experience.	5. Decision making is based on evidence.
6. "Do no harm" is an individual responsibility.	6. Safety is a system property.
7. Secrecy is necessary.	7. Transparency is necessary.
8. The system reacts to needs.	8. Needs are anticipated.
9. Cost reduction is sought.	9. Waste is continuously decreased.
10. Preference is given to professional roles over the system.	10. Cooperation among clinicians is a priority.

The organization viewed as a system in Figure 6.2 provides a generic, conceptual model of a linkage of processes for any organization. Sometimes it is useful to develop a specific conceptual model of the organization before listing processes to build the linkage of processes. This is particularly true for a large organization with multiple business units, regions, and locations. Particular departments may benefit by first developing a more specific conceptual view of how its area fits into the rest of the organization.

Some organizations find it helpful to prepare a conceptual diagram of the organization as a system. The idea is to redraw the organization viewed as a system (see Figure 6.2) with labels that fit your organization.

Dr. Rachel Dali commented at this point in the discussion, "Dr. Chow, I think I have just learned something important about our responsibilities as a leadership team. From your presentation, it is apparent to me that this leadership team not only has ownership of many of the delivery system processes, but we also have great responsibilities in what you are calling the driver processes. Is my view correct?" Dr. Chow responded, "Absolutely, Dr. Dali. These processes are very important and help to influence and align the rest of the system." Dr. Dali added, "I am a little concerned that our driver work processes might not be as defined as the delivery system processes." At this point several leaders concurred. Dr. Tan joked, "This might be why we don't have our board entirely focused." After some chuckles, Dr. Chow added, "These are excellent observations. The board is a governing body whose processes all reside in the drivers since they influence and ensure that we are aligned to our purpose. As a leadership team, we can help our board be more effective, if we can define their role and driver processes. Let's continue with how to define our system, keeping in mind that each of us understands our part of the system as it exists today. As we share, we will be learning and recognizing as a team how the system actually works."

Defining the System

Defining the boundary of your system is important, because the boundary differentiates the system from other systems. This boundary provides focus, helps to define important relationships, and helps leaders to identify potential partners internal and external to your organization.

Boundaries may be physical or mental. Like a fence around a yard, the boundary separates the system from others. Managing the "gates in the fence" (the openings that allow interactions with the environment outside the system) is an important part of optimizing the system.

When developing a systems view, where should we draw the boundaries? Ideally we should view the entire organization as one system and focus on optimizing that system. For many larger organizations, this approach leads to levels of complexity that can overwhelm any type of study and analysis. Can this large organization be broken into parts that are more manageable? Not if they are interdependent.

But there may be ways to divide the organization into smaller systems to help reduce complexity and retain the concept of a system. The focus then becomes optimizing the smaller systems created by the division. Examples of dividing the organization into smaller parts include types of health care units focused on different markets or regions that operate in different geographic areas.

When establishing satellite systems, the following principles are guidelines based on systems thinking:

1. Each satellite system should connect directly to an external customer (patient).
2. Each satellite system should be as independent as possible from the other satellite systems. Although some dependence will usually exist, no part should have to depend on another part to accomplish its purpose.
3. Each satellite system should contain all of the important functions needed to accomplish its purpose. Any support needed from the parent organization, or from other satellites, should be formally treated as support from an external supplier.

Each of the organization's satellites needs a statement of purpose, consistent with the purpose of the larger organization. Mayo's different clinics are a good example of multiple systems with the same purpose and philosophy.

In a health services organization with multiple medical centers, clinics, hospitals, and laboratories, systems could be defined by geographic location. Each unit (hospital, clinic, and laboratory) would be part of a satellite system defined to serve a particular community. All the necessary functions of the service would be available in each unit. The parent organization would provide necessary administrative services not contained in any of the satellites (see Figure 6.9 for an example of applying this logic).

In each of these examples, the satellites of the health care organization can work relatively independently. It is an important part of the leader's job to ensure that no competition arises between satellites that are serving patients and families. Another important part of the leader's work is to form internal partnerships to move all the parts of the organization from independence to collaboration.

Figure 6.9 Defining the Satellites of the System for a Health Services Organization

System 1: Four Hospitals, Six Clinics, with Administration as a Supplier

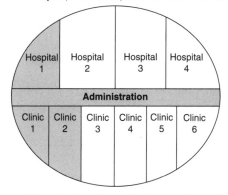

System 2: One Hospital, Two Clinics, with Administration as a Supplier

System 3: Two Hospitals, Administration, and Three Clinics

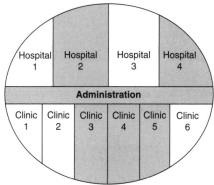

Source: Quality as a Business Strategy (Austin, TX: API-Austin, 1998). Available online from http://www.pipproducts.com/books.html.

Dr. Chow finished the exercise of drawing boundaries of the system for the leadership team. He then outlined a generic view of the health care system (found in Chapter 11) and detailed examples from Jönköping County Council, a dialysis clinic viewed as a system, and OCHIN. (See Chapter 10 for these examples). Dr. Tan summarized, "From Dr. Chow's presentation it is apparent we have some work to do as a leadership team. Dr. Chow, what is our next step?" Dr. Chow replied, "At our next meeting let's create the conceptual view of our system given the boundaries we defined today. From that we can begin the detailed work." Dr. Tan and the leadership team thanked Dr. Chow for a very informative presentation. Dr. Tan said she was looking forward to their next meeting and the others agreed.

Why Systems Thinking Is Difficult

Since Newton published *Mathematical Principles of Natural Philosophy* in 1687, the method of inquiry in the West has been dominated by *analysis*. All of us have been taught the analytical method of solving a problem. We must still analyze and solve problems, but increases in complexity and interdependence demand that we now learn to make improvements with *systems thinking*. We may not get a real improvement for our organization by solving a problem in one department that does not optimize the whole system.

With analysis, the objective is to understand how something works. First we break it down into parts, study each of the parts independently, and then put it back together. The result is *knowledge* of *how* the parts fit together. Solving problems with systems thinking begins and ends with an understanding of how the whole interacts with its environment and how its parts interact to achieve a purpose. Systems thinking helps us *understand why* something works as it does. The study of systems requires a new vocabulary and set of thought processes, understanding the interaction of the parts and the detail of the parts, while understanding the whole. Table 6.2 compares the steps of analysis with systems thinking.

Table 6.2 Comparison of Analysis and Systems Thinking

Method of Inquiry	Analysis	Systems Thinking
First Stage	Break into parts the whole which is to be explained	System is identified and considered as a whole (Synthesis)
Second Stage	Explanations are made for each part separately (Analysis)	Explanations are made concerning the whole (Analysis)
Third Stage	Explanations are then taken together to explain the whole (Synthesis)	Behavior of the subsystems are explained in terms of their role or function within the whole (Synthesis)
Focus	Structure (Internal)	Function (External)
Question Answered	How do things work?	Why do things operate as they do?
Result	Knowledge (Describe)	Understanding (Explain)

Changing a System

Two basic types of change of a system are[4]

- **Reactive change:** A change that reacts to process within a part of the system that does not change the other parts or the system as a whole. This includes routine changes required to keep the organization running. Reactive changes can be characterized by the following attributes:
  - Solve problems or react
  - Return the system to prior condition
  - Tradeoff among measures, increasing quality while increasing costs
  - Short-term impact
- **Fundamental change:** Transforming the system, which can involve changing its purpose or its parts in a way that changes how system components interact to produce results. Fundamental changes include the following:
  - Design or redesign of some aspect of the system
  - Necessary for improvement beyond problems

- Fundamentally alters the system and what people do
- Impacts several measures in a positive direction, increasing quality while also reducing costs
- Long-term impact

Leverage, Constraints, and Bottlenecks

To optimize the system to achieve its purpose, the components of the system must be continuously designed and redesigned. These efforts of an organization should be focused to have the biggest impact on the system. Another important concept from systems thinking is the idea of **leverage**, meaning that some small, very specific actions can produce significant changes in the system.

A **constraint**, or **bottleneck**, can be anything that restricts the throughput of a system. A constraint within an organization can be any resource where the demand for that resource is greater than its available capacity. In order to increase the throughput in a system, the constraints should be identified, exploited if possible, and removed if necessary. It is often difficult to identify a constraint by evaluating the demand and the capacity for each resource. As an alternative, look for certain signals within the system. Where is material or information in short supply? Where are the largest waiting times to use a resource? Where is inventory stacking up? These signals will serve as aids in identifying a constraint.

Once a constraint is identified, it should be studied to learn if any of the capacity of the resource is being wasted. Goldratt refers to this as exploiting the constraint.[5] Because a constraint determines the capacity of the system, it should never be idle. Resources that are not constraints may have idle time as the flow through the system will be determined by the flow through the constraint. Therefore, these resources may be able to take some of the load off the constraint.

To focus on improvement through the removal of constraints, Goldratt recommends the following five steps:[6]

1. Identify the system's constraints (prioritize all constraints according to their impact on the goal).
2. Decide how to exploit the system's constraints (manage all other resources to supply all that the constraints will consume).
3. Subordinate everything else to the decisions in Step 2.

4. Elevate the constraints of the system.
5. If a constraint is broken in the previous steps, go back to Step 1.

As an example, a hospital's lack of operating rooms was forcing some physicians to move their operations to other hospitals. When the hospital staff began to study the situation, they found that lack of operating rooms was a constraint only in the morning hours. This was the time desired by most physicians and patients. The hospital began to exploit this constraint by allowing patients who were willing to have their operations scheduled in the afternoon to check in on that day rather than the night before. This eliminated a night's stay in the hospital and increased the number of patients who were willing to have their operations in the afternoon. In addition, physicians were given a lower rate for use of operating rooms in the afternoon.

Dr. Rachel Dali observed, "Before we had a systems view, when we would discuss problems, the conversation usually turned to who did that? Now it seems we are asking deeper questions about the work processes, bottlenecks, and reactive versus fundamental changes." Dr. Chow was enthused by the shared learning of the team and explained, "Without a systems view, we can only see the people in the system, ignoring the processes which make up the system. When things go wrong, it is easier to attribute blame to people we see rather than the processes they use. During our Improvement Professional workshop on systems, we learned that Dr. Deming observed that 94 percent of the problems are due to the system—not people—behaving badly. As a leadership team, we now have the system and the associated processes under suspicion and are asking different questions as leaders." Dr. Tan, the CEO, was very pleased with the learning and cooperation during these discussions; gone was the typical blame and defensiveness. Dr. Tan added, "I think we have taken a great step to becoming a learning organization. I can see it in the questions and the way we handle challenges. Thanks, Dr. Chow, for your guidance and help."

After learning about the constraint on preferred times to operate, the hospital staff turned their attention to improving patient satisfaction. The leadership team completed the conceptual and detailed views of their health care system. The hospital staff began using the systems map to highlight several processes that are key patient and family contacts where they can improve their patient satisfaction scores. The systems view was also used in meetings to discuss issues and problems.

Systems and People: Improving Behavior

A serious challenge in many health care organizations is avoiding mistakes that can harm patients. Often the people who make the mistakes are blamed when in fact the fault lies mainly in processes and interdependencies within the system.

Attribution theory describes the tendency for observers to underestimate situational (the system) influences and overestimate individual motives and personality traits as the cause of behavior. Deming wrote, "A fault in the interpretation of observations, seen everywhere, is to suppose that every event (defect, mistake, accident) is attributable to someone (usually the one nearest at hand), or is related to some special event. The fact is most troubles with service and production lie in the system."[7]

For example, in one health care system operating room nurses sometimes made mistakes because each surgeon used different processes for preparing patients. Nurses had a difficult time keeping track of the various processes used by different surgeons. When surgeons and nurses were able to agree on a common process, mistakes were no longer made.

To fundamentally change a health care system, you need to engage the system's leaders in understanding the need for change and how a changed system would improve future results. Resistance to change may be based on concern about future roles or beliefs and the insistence that what worked in the past should be maintained. Leaders need to surface these views and explain why implementing the changes that will achieve the vision will improve health outcomes and service quality while reducing cost. Leaders must do the following:

- Celebrate and bury the past
- Build the will to change the present
- Define a positive vision for the future

Leaders need to develop a communication plan to explain why what worked in the past no longer applies, why the challenges of the present require our attention and must be changed, and how future challenge will be addressed by the changes realized by the idealized vision of the system.

Intermountain (IHC) uses data to deal with resistance in the system. Health care professionals are shown which procedures bring the best results. Rather than creating conflict, IHC leaders communicate the results so that everyone can learn what works. Furthermore, the evidence-based procedures are built into the information system and work processes; health care professionals must either follow them or actively modify them.

Because changes in processes require changes in roles and relationships, training is usually needed. How can we measure the value of training? The immediate results may be higher costs and lower productivity. Investment in training depends on a belief in the organization's future. In contrast to investments like training where the benefits will only be seen in the long run, some actions produce immediate gains but long-term difficulties. An example might be what we have defined as a *reactive change* in this chapter: laying off people to reduce costs at the expense of service quality. Current problems in a system are usually the result of yesterday's solutions to problems where the system no longer meets the changing demands of society and customers. *Fundamental changes* to the system can result in improved patient outcomes, reduced per capita costs, and improvement of population health. When focused on improvement of a system our changes need not result in a zero-sum game; it is possible to improve care while lowering costs.

A system cannot be transformed all at once. Chapter 10 presents several case studies which each show how a systems view was used to help develop a vision of an organizational system. Conceptual views of the system are used to make a detailed linkage of processes that together work to achieve the organization's purpose. By showing these processes, you help your people and collaborators to understand the interdependencies in the organization and to focus on the needs of internal as well as external customers.

The other is the set of measures of the organizational system. This serves as an indicator of the present performance of the system and can be used to predict how the transformed system will perform. Using the theory of variation presented in Chapter 7 to more effectively respond to patterns of variation will be essential; which patterns of variation tell us that the pattern is "common" to the current system and must be changed fundamentally? Which patterns of variation tell us that the variation is due to special circumstances and that we may be able to learn from this variation immediately by reacting?

It takes time to change a system. In Chapter 11, we describe a method to develop a five-year plan to implement a vision of an ideal organization using the Four Ps discussed in this chapter.

SUMMARY

The following key points have been discussed in this chapter:

- Definition of a system with the Four Ps as a foundation: a collection of interdependent *processes* and other elements with *people* working interactively guided by *practical values* to accomplish the *purpose* of the system.
- Transforming the organization means moving from the organizational chart view to viewing the organization as a system.
- Deming's organization viewed as a system can be used as a template to develop a conceptual view of your system. Using Deming's diagram there are three types of processes:
  - Mainstay: defines the delivery system processes that impact the patient
  - Driver: processes that can change how we operate the system
  - Support: processes that are essential to carry out the mainstay and driver processes
- Systems are made up of work processes. All work is a process. Understanding work as a process is an essential skill for everyone in the system.
- When making changes it is essential to understand the difference between detail and dynamic complexity.
- Leaders need to appreciate the difference between analysis and systems thinking. Systems thinking involves the role of synthesis and consideration of the whole system before attempting analysis.
- The attribution error can lead to blaming people for systemic causes.

KEY TERMS

Attribution theory

Bottleneck

Complex adaptive systems

Constraint

Detailed complexity

Driver processes

Dynamic complexity

Fundamental change

Interdependence

Key process

Leverage

Linkage of processes

Mainstay processes

Reactive change

Support processes

Systems thinking

EXERCISES

The following exercises can help you to think about your organization as a system and what it takes to develop it into a learning organization.

1. Draw a conceptual view of your organization viewed as a system. Using Figure 6.2 as a guideline, draw your organization's version of the organization as a system. See Chapter 10 case studies for various examples of systems diagrams.
2. Draw a large circle to describe your entire organization. Show the various parts (regions, departments, offices, staffs, projects, and so on) in your organization. See Figure 6.9 for an example.
3. Considering your organization, divide the organization into parts so that each part can be treated as a separate system. Draw a picture of the total organization and the systems in the organization. See Figure 6.9.

4. Describe some key leverage points in your organization. Describe some constraints or bottlenecks in your organization. Describe a change that could potentially eliminate these constraints.

5. Describe a recent situation in which you may have committed the fundamental attribution error.

6. Describe an example of a change in your organization that resulted in a noticeable change in the behavior of the employees.

7. Earlier in the chapter we discussed the Four Ps. Consider the questions below relative to your system:

- Purpose:
  - What is the purpose of our organization?
  - Who are we serving?
  - What value do we add for them?
  - What do we measure that tells us we are accomplishing our purpose?
- Processes:
  - How are our work processes linked to make the system achieve its purpose effectively and efficiently?
  - What 20 percent of the processes do we depend upon to accomplish our purpose?
- People:
  - What are the *roles* and *responsibilities* we need to fill and what kinds of people do we need to fill them?
  - What are the skills they need to have?
  - How should they interact? What are the important *relationships*?
  - What kinds of personality traits are we looking for?
  - What kinds of relationships do we need to manage?
  - What *rewards* are essential for our people?
  - How should we *recognize* contributions to the organization?
- Practical Values:
  - What are the practical values that ensure we achieve the system's purpose?
  - How do we respond when one of those values is not practiced?

8. Consider the conceptual view of a healthcare system that is described in Figure 6.10.

- In what ways would your health care system be similar to the subsystems in this diagram?
- In what ways would your system be different?

Figure 6.10   Conceptual View of a Health Care System

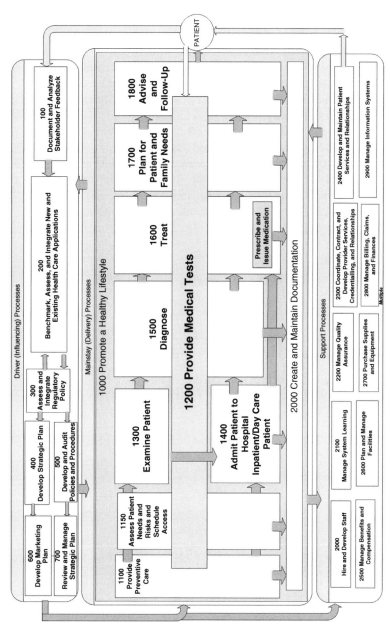

ENDNOTES

1. Dr. W. Edwards Deming developed his famous 14 points that were taught in his four-day seminars. Point #1: Create constancy of purpose toward improvement of product and service, with the aim to become competitive and to stay in business, and to provide jobs. W. Edwards Deming, *Out of the Crisis* (Cambridge, MA: MIT Press, 2011), Kindle edition, p. 23.
2. Michael Porter, *The Competitive Advantage of Nations* (New York: The Free Press, 1990).
3. Institute of Medicine, *Crossing the Quality Chasm: A New Health System for the 21st Century* (Washington, DC: National Academy Press, 2001).
4. Gerald J. Langley, Ronald D. Moen, Kevin M. Nolan, Thomas W. Nolan, Clifford L. Norman, and Lloyd P. Provost, *The Improvement Guide: A Practical Approach to Enhancing Organizational Performance* (San Francisco: Jossey-Bass, 2009), Kindle edition, loc. 2244–2245.
5. Eliyahu Goldratt and Jeff Cox, *The Goal* (New York: North River Press, 1986).
6. Ibid., 301.
7. W. Edwards Deming, *Out of the Crisis* (Cambridge, MA: MIT Press, 2011), Kindle edition, p. 314.

STATISTICAL THINKING FOR HEALTH CARE LEADERS

Knowledge About Variation

Robert Davis, vice president of human resources for his health care organization, had recently attended a workshop called "Profound Knowledge for Leaders." Bob found learning about systems, psychology, and theory of knowledge extremely informative. But he felt he had not fully understood statistical thinking. When he returned to his organization, a health care system in the Midwest, he called Kerri Barnett, one of the improvement professionals in his organization. Kerri was currently leading eleven projects inside the organization. When Kerri arrived at the office, Bob expressed his concern with the recent workshop: "Kerri, I have just spent the last two days learning about the system of profound knowledge. I really enjoyed the discussion around everything except the theory of variation. Frankly, it was challenging. In my MBA education, we were taught about managing exceptions and variances and I thought I understood how to use data in making decisions. But from this experience, I think I may be making mistakes. Would you mind giving me a little coaching?" Kerri smiled, "Not at all, Bob, it would be my pleasure."

The success of a learning organization will be determined by specific measurements of cost and quality, safety and efficiency. A systemic vision includes not only how people will work together, but also how processes and systems will be designed and continually improved. This requires knowledge of variation and statistics.[1]

Leaders use statistics to test processes and make predictions about interventions. Have our efforts reduced infection rates? Do the two medication errors indicate a negative trend? Was the improved performance this week the result of the changes we made? Or was it just luck? The ability to improve processes to strengthen organizational purpose requires the ability to answer questions like these. And that requires knowledge of variation and statistics.

An improvement team in a major health system was convinced that doctors were a major problem relative to having positive intervention scores on patient surveys. The leader of the improvement team collected 20–100 surveys (average sample size was approximately 60 surveys) for each doctor. Figure 7.1 describes the control chart for percentage of surveys that indicated a positive intervention from the viewpoint of the patient.

What are we to conclude from these data? Which doctors should we question? Later in the chapter we will address these questions, but for now let's consider the important ideas that underlie this important tool.

One of the pioneers in developing the theory to understand variation was Walter A. Shewhart. His work dates back to the 1920s.

Figure 7.1   Control Chart for Positive Intervention by Doctor

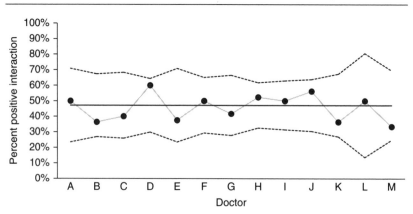

When plotting data over time, Shewhart observed two situations: (1) in some cases the pattern in the data were predictable and (2) in other cases it was unpredictable. Based on these observations, Shewhart used statistical theory to develop a means of understanding variation in systems based on patterns of variation over time. His method is based on the following definitions (first introduced in Chapter 5):[2]

- **Common causes:** those causes inherent in the process (or system) over time that affect everyone working in the process and all outcomes of the process
- **Special causes:** those causes *not* part of the process (or system) all the time or that do not affect everyone, but which arise because of specific circumstances

A system that has only common causes affecting the outcomes is called a **stable system**, or one that is in a state of **statistical control**. A stable process implies only that the variation is **predictable** within statistically established limits. A system whose outcomes are affected by both common causes and special causes is called an **unstable system**. An unstable system does not necessarily mean one with large variation. It means that the magnitude of the variation from one time period to the next is unpredictable.

Besides providing these basic concepts of variation, Shewhart also provided the method for determining whether a system is dominated by common or special causes. This method is called the Shewhart Control Chart. The **control chart** is a statistical tool used to distinguish between variation in a measure of quality due to common causes and variation due to special causes. The name used to describe the chart ("control") is misleading, as the most common uses of these charts are to learn about variation and to evaluate the impact of changes. A better name might be "learning charts." But the name Shewhart chose for the chart in the 1920s has persisted. Our example in Figure 7.1 is an example of a control chart.

The construction of a control chart typically involves

- Plotting the data or some summary of the data in a run order (time is the most common order)
- Determining some measure of the central tendency of the data (such as the average)

- Determining some measure of the common cause variation of the data
- Calculating a centerline and upper and lower **control limits** (see Figure 7.1)

Kerri and Bob met the next day at lunch. Kerri explained that understanding the difference between special and common cause variation was at the heart of understanding data for decision making. Kerri said, "Understanding the difference tells you when to react and when not to react. This knowledge saves your valuable time. The control chart method helps us to understand if results are caused by special causes or common causes." Bob then asked, "So understanding the special cause pattern is important. Won't the computer do that for me?" Kerri responded, "Bob there are software packages that will highlight special causes, but it is not necessary to use them. There are only five basic patterns and you can commit these to memory." Bob said, "Kerri, this is great—do you have some time tomorrow?" Kerri was very pleased with Bob's eagerness to learn about variation and readily agreed to another meeting.

Interpretation of a Control Chart

The control chart provides a basis for taking action to improve a process. A process is considered to be stable when there is a random distribution of the plotted points within the control limits. For a stable process, action should be directed at identifying the important causes of variation common to all of the points. If the distribution (or pattern) of points is not random, the process is considered to be unstable and action should be taken to learn about the special causes of variation.

There is general agreement among users of control charts that a single point outside the control limits is an indication of a special cause of variation. However, there have been many suggestions for systems of **rules to identify special causes** which appear as nonrandom patterns within the control limits. Figure 7.2 contains five rules for identifying special causes that are recommended for use with control charts.

A process that has only common causes affecting the outcomes is called a *stable* process, or one that is in a state of *statistical control*.

Figure 7.2 Rules for Determining a Special Cause

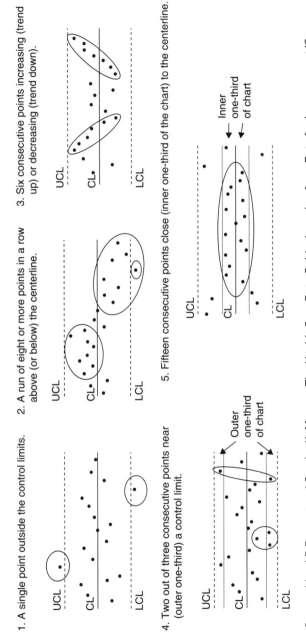

1. A single point outside the control limits.

2. A run of eight or more points in a row above (or below) the centerline.

3. Six consecutive points increasing (trend up) or decreasing (trend down).

4. Two out of three consecutive points near (outer one-third) a control limit.

5. Fifteen consecutive points close (inner one-third of the chart) to the centerline.

Source: Lloyd P. Provost and Sandra K. Murray, *The Health Care Data Guide: Learning from Data for Improvement* (San Francisco: Jossey-Bass, 2011).

In a stable process, the causal system of variation remains essentially constant over time. This does not mean that there is no variation in the outcomes of the process, that the variation is small, or that outcomes meet requirements. It only implies that the variation is predictable within statistically established limits. In practice, this indicates that a fundamental change to the system is needed for improvement.

A process whose outcomes are affected by both common and special causes of variation is called an *unstable* process. An unstable process is not necessarily one with large variation. Rather, the magnitude of variation from one period to the next is unpredictable. If special causes can be identified and removed, the process becomes stable. Its performance becomes predictable. In practical terms this implies that improvement can occur by identifying the special causes and taking appropriate action.

> After Kerri described the five basic patterns for control charts, she said, "Bob, there are some other guidelines we use when applying the five special cause rules." Bob's hopes for simplicity beginning to dim, he said, "Kerri, I had a feeling it was going to get more complicated—you are going to have to help me through this!" Assuring Bob that they were pretty straightforward, Kerri then stated the guidelines for using the special cause rules.

When applying the rules, the following guidelines will help with consistent interpretation of charts:

- Ties between two consecutive points do not cancel or add to a trend (rule 3).
- A point exactly on a control limit is not considered outside the limit (rule 1).
- When control charts have varying limits due to varying numbers of measurements within subgroups, then rule 3 should not be applied.
- A point exactly on the centerline does not cancel or count toward a run (rule 2).
- When there is not a lower or upper control limit (for example, on a range chart with less than seven measures in a subgroup or on a process chart with 100 percent as a possible result for the process), rules 1 and 4 do not apply to the missing limit.

Given our rules for identifying special causes, consider our first example of the control chart with positive intervention scores. We posed these questions:

- What are we to conclude from these data?
- Which doctors should we question?

From applying the rules for special causes in Figure 7.2, it appears that we have no special causes in the control chart depicted in Figure 7.1. We would say that the process is dominated by common cause variation. In fact, the system is producing patient satisfaction with interventions at 47 percent. To make improvements in this process something fundamental must be changed in the system that is currently being used to interact with the patients.

> During their lunch discussions, Kerri had shown Bob the same chart on the positive interactions. She then asked Bob, "Which doctors should we be talking to, given what we have learned about special causes?" Bob answered, "Kerri, two days ago, I would have scheduled appointments with those who were below average, or about half of them." Kerri and Bob laughed together.

Typical responses are to blame the doctors for the problems or to exhort them to be more patient-focused and have a better bedside manner. These could be issues, but whatever they are, they are common to the system. Another popular but equally demotivating approach is to congratulate the doctors who are above average and reprimand those who are below average. It should come as no surprise to anyone that about half of the doctors will be below and half above average. Taking any of the typical approaches would alienate the doctors who are probably doing their best under the current system. We need another approach with statistical thinking.

In this approach, we would want to involve the doctors in developing, testing, and implementing changes to improve the patient experience. Their intimate knowledge of the process would be essential to the improvement effort. People are generally motivated to participate in improving processes that influence their work. Participation increases their sense of responsibility and clarifies the reasons for the process. When a leader of a learning organization uses an understanding of variation to create the opportunity for learning, this demonstrates that the leader is more interested in creating a learning organization than in finding fault.

We pointed out that nurses at an operating room at a hospital traced errors to confusion caused by fifteen different protocols of surgeons. Once the surgeons and nurses developed and agreed to a common protocol, errors disappeared.

Avoiding the Two Kinds of Mistakes in Reacting to Variation

In developing the control chart method, Shewhart emphasized the importance of not looking for special causes when they do not exist and overlooking special causes that do exist. Table 7.1 illustrates the impact of the two mistakes that result in unnecessary costs: **mistake 1—type 1 error**, looking for trouble when nothing has changed; and **mistake 2—type 2 error**, not taking action when in fact we have some opportunities to learn. The other two quadrants indicate correct decisions. When the actual situation (see A) has changed and we react to it as special, we are most likely to learn with profit. When there is no change in the real world and we treat it as common cause variation, again we have acted properly (see B) and we have learned with profit. Our aim in understanding the difference between special and common cause variation is minimize the opportunities for overreacting and underreacting to mistakes 1 and 2.

Table 7.1   Mistakes Made in Attempts to Improve Results

Mistake 1: React to an outcome as if it came from a special cause, when actually it came from common causes of variation.

Mistake 2: Treat an outcome as if it came from common causes of variation, when actually it came from a special cause.

	Actual Situation of System	
Action	**No Change**	**Change**
Take action on individual outcome; Treat as a *special cause variation*.	− $ Mistake 1	+ $ Correct Decision (A)
Treat outcome as part of system; work on changing the system-Treat as *common cause variation*.	+ $ Correct Decision (B)	− $ Mistake 2

At their next meeting, Bob had a question. "Kerri, what are the control limits based upon?" Kerri described the underlying rationale that Shewhart used to establish control limits. Kerri explained, "The main idea was to be able to find special causes when they occurred so the user could learn and not waste time looking for issues when there was nothing to learn." Bob commented, "This would seem to be a valuable tool for leaders when we are reviewing the hospital dashboard. Why don't we discuss that at our next meeting? I will send you a copy with the data." Kerri felt this would be a big step forward, not only for Bob, but for other leaders who are stretched for time. Kerri said, "Let's get back your question on the rationale behind the Shewhart limits on the control chart."

Shewhart provided a rationale for the use of the control chart and the corresponding three-sigma limits:

- The limits have a basis in statistical theory.
- The limits have proven in practice to distinguish between special and common causes of variation.
- In most cases, use of the limits will approximately minimize the total cost due to overreaction and underreaction to variation in the process.
- The limits protect the morale of workers in the process by defining the magnitude of the variation that has been built into the process.

Graphical Display Using Statistical Thinking

As a leader in health care, you have probably been exposed to the **dashboard** idea of looking at measures. Figure 7.3 provides an example that describes sixteen key measures for a hospital that have been grouped into the following categories:

- Patient perspective
- Patient safety
- Clinical
- Employee perspective
- Operational performance
- Community perspective
- Financial perspective

Figure 7.3   Hospital Dashboard[3]

Traffic Light Legend: ◯ Red

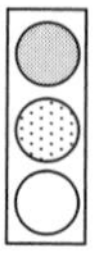

◯ Yellow

◯ Green

Measurement Category	Hospital System Level Goals and Measures						
	FY 2009 Goal	Long-Term Goal	FY 2007	FY 2008	FY 2009 QI	FY 2009 Q2	FY 2009 Q3
Patients							
1. Overall Satification Rating: Percent who would recommend (includes inpatient, outpatient, ED and Home Health)	60.00%	80.00%	37.98%	48.98%	57.19%	56.25%	51.69%
2. Wait Time for 3rd Next Available Appt: Percent of areas with appointment available in less than or equal to 7 business days.	65.0%	100.0%	53.5%	54.3%	54.3%	61.2%	65.1%
Patient Safety							
3. Safety Events per 10,000 Adjusted Days	0.28	0.20	0.35	0.31	0.31	0.30	0.28
4. Percent Mortality	3.60	3.00	4.00	4.00	3.48	3.50	3.42
5. Infections per 1,000 Patient Days	2.00	0.00	3.37	4.33	4.39	2.58	1.96
Clinical							
6. Percent Unplanned Readmissions	3.50%	1.50%	6.10%	4.80%	4.60%	4.10%	3.50%
7. Percent Eligible Patients Receiving Perfect Care Evidence Based Care (Inpatient and ED)	95.0%	100.0%	46.0%	74.1%	88.0%	91.7%	88.7%
Employees							
8. Percent Voluntary Employee Turnover	5.80%	5.20%	5.20%	6.38%	6.10%	6.33%	6.30%
9. Employee Satisfaction: Average rating (1–5 Scale) 5 Best	4	4.25	3.9	3.8	3.96	3.98	3.96
Operational Performance							
10. Percent Occupancy	88.0%	90.0%	81.3%	84.0%	91.3%	85.6%	87.2%
11. Average Length of Stay (LOS)	4.3	3.8	5.2	4.9	4.6	4.7	4.3
12. Physician Satisfaction: Average rating (1–5 scale)	4	4.25	3.8	3.84	3.96	3.8	3.87
Community							
13. Percent of Budget Allocated to Non-recompensed Care	7.00%	7.00%	5.91%	7.00%	6.90%	6.93%	7.00%
14. Percent of Budget Spent on Community Health Promotion Programs	0.30%	0.30%	0.32%	0.29%	0.28%	0.31%	0.29%
Financial							
15. Operating Margin Percent	1.20%	1.50%	-0.50%	0.70%	0.90%	0.40%	0.70%
16. Monthly Revenue (Million)	20	20.6	17.6	16.9	17.5	18.3	19.2

For each measure the annual goal is displayed along with comparison of two prior years. For the current year of 2009, we also provide the quarterly results. To make the analysis quick and easy the use of traffic lights are used. Green is good, yellow is caution, and red means attention is needed ... now! This method is very popular. But what are we losing by using it? Let's consider the data in view of the theory of variation and statistical thinking.

Bob showed up at lunch ready to discuss the hospital dashboard with Kerri. "Good afternoon Kerri, did you have time to look at our dashboard?" "Yes, I did and I have prepared some charts to compare the dashboard with signals on the control charts. How does the leadership team use this report Bob?" Bob responded, "It is pretty straightforward—anything in red has to be explained. The executive responsible for the red light is required to explain the cause. What did you learn from looking at the control charts?" Kerri said, "Given your learning about the theory of variation I think you might have some other ideas about how the executive team should respond to variation." Bob said, "Good, let's get started."

Figure 7.4 highlights measure number 3, Safety Events per 10,000 Adjusted Patient Days. The goal for FY 2009 is 0.28 Events per 10,000 Adjusted Patient Days. The long-term goal is 0.20. In FY 2007 the actual was 0.35, FY 2008 was 0.31. The quarters for 2009 are displayed as follows:

FY 2009 Q1	0.31	Red
FY 2009 Q2	0.30	Red
FY 2009 Q3	0.28	Green

So what are we losing with this display? As the leader you certainly would like to know if this happy news is from stable data and predictable for the future. How do we know? From this information we do not know. This could be a trend of one. The only method that permits us to make a prediction and understand stability relative to a measure is the

Figure 7.4   Safety Events per 10,000 Adjusted Patient Days

Patients	FY 09 Goal	Long Term Goal	FY 2007	FY 2008	FY 2009 Q1	FY 2009 Q2	FY 2009 Q3
3. Safety Events per 10,000 Adjusted Bed Days	0.28	0.20	0.35	0.31	0.31	0.30	0.28

Figure 7.5　Safety Events per 10,000 Adjusted Patient Days: Control Chart

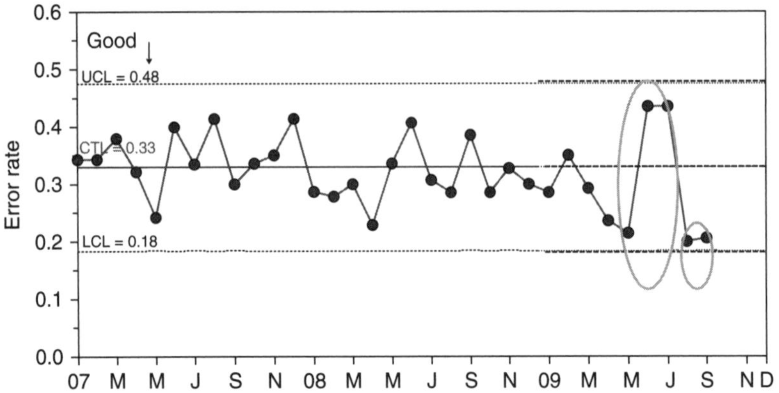

Shewhart Control Chart. Figure 7.5 describes the control chart for data being reported in our dashboard.

What are we learning from the control chart? Is the process stable? To answer this question, we can refer to the special cause signals described in Figure 7.2. Rule number 4 is present starting in May and continuing through September 2009. The data is showing us that safety events per 10,000 adjusted patient days is not predictable. If the last two data points were the result of a predicted improvement, then we can be very happy about our green dashboard. If we do not have knowledge of the special causes, then our ability to predict the future has been greatly diminished.

As we are performing better than our goal, what is the problem? Consider the control chart in Figure 7.6 concerning the rate of unplanned returns to the emergency department. Our goal is 7.5 or less per 1,000 discharges. We have not had a month worse than that figure for nineteen months! What does the control chart show that might cause us to be concerned? Referring to the five special cause rules in Figure 7.2, we can see that we have a statistical signal in our data in the form of the "trend rule." Our control chart is unstable. We have something to learn; this special cause must be investigated not only to avert going above our stated goal, but, more important, to learn how we might improve. If this measure were on our dashboard, it would be showing green because we are below goal. In fact, a more useful engagement of the lights on a dashboard would show this signal as red.

Figure 7.6   Control Chart of Unplanned Returns
to the Emergency Department

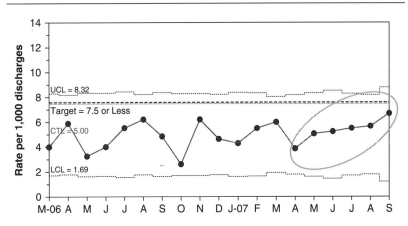

Consider the control chart in Figure 7.7 on infections per 1,000 patient days. We have preserved the traffic signal color patterns on the table to the left of the graphic. When you consider the control chart relative to the

Figure 7.7   Infections per 1,000 Patient Days: Total

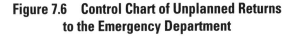

presence of special causes, we have no patterns. However, we do have all the colors of the traffic lights changing over time. None of this would be bad if the changing colors did not lead to wasted efforts. In fact, we are making mistakes one and two from Table 7.1. We are overreacting to common cause variation with red and yellow lights.

Because common cause variation is exhibited in the control chart, the leaders have wasted time either exhorting people to take action or celebrating green lights. Deming referred to reacting to common cause variation without knowledge as tampering. Better practice would use the theory of variation, convene a team of people with knowledge, and determine how we are going to reduce infections per 1,000 patient days.

When using a dashboard to analyze the data from your system, it is essential to use statistical thinking to analyze the data. Using statistical thinking is important to properly develop learning from data that contribute to the ability of the leader to engage in productive foresight.

As their lunch discussion was winding down, Kerri asked Bob, "What are you learning, Bob, about the dashboard, traffic lights, and the use of control charts?" "Kerri, I am going to have to give this some thought. I really like the idea of seeing the measures on one page. But I can also see the folly of creating one or both of the mistakes you mentioned earlier: overreacting and wasting time or underreacting and not learning. This concerns me. What if we had the traffic signals connected to the special cause rules instead of goals?" Kerri responded, "Bob, that would be a step in the right direction. Adding the data on control charts or even **run charts** would be useful." "Kerri, we haven't talked about run charts. Can we discuss these charts at our meeting this Friday?" Bob said. Kerri made a note to bring her material on run charts for the next meeting. "See you on Friday, Bob!"

Power of Simple Run Charts for Data Display

To reduce infections and other side effects, hospitals are trying to minimize the number of days an intensive care patient has to spend on a mechanical ventilator. The ICU director in one hospital was asked to investigate why the vent days per patient were high in the last quarter's management report. In August, she put together an improvement team that investigated and learned that some of the standard procedures were not being followed. The team conducted staff training to review the standard procedures and by the end of the year reported a 50 percent reduction in average ventilator days in the unit, with the rate now running below the goal of four days. Figure 7.8[4] shows a run chart the quality improvement (QI) team used to report their results. What would be your assessment of the work of the QI team and the changes started in August, 2003, described in Figure 7.9. Have they made an improvement? Let's consider more about variation before returning to this question.

Figure 7.8   Reduction in Average Ventilator Days

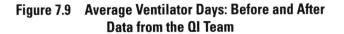

Figure 7.9   Average Ventilator Days: Before and After Data from the QI Team

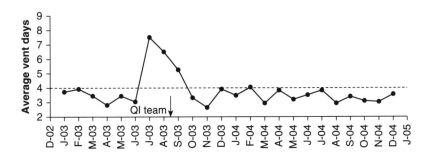

Figure 7.10   Using Bar Charts to Compare Before and After

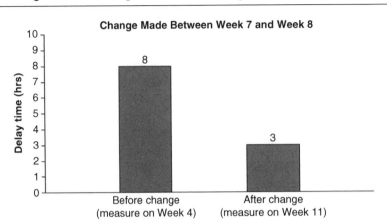

At the end of the year, the management team was reviewing the annual performance and noticed that the average of the ventilator days was not much different from the previous two years. They were concerned that the days had crept back up after the QI team's work. They prepared a run chart of the last two years to better understand what was going on. This second run chart showed that the system had deviated from its expected performance in July 2003, and the work of the QI team brought the performance back to norm (a reactive change). Monitoring processes and reacting to deviations in performance are important components of effective quality control in any organization, but not the same as improving the system by making a fundamental change.

Once a change is made, continuing to plot data over time and observe the patterns helps to determine whether the change is an improvement. Consider Figure 7.10. Would you say that the change being made between weeks 7 and 8 had made an improvement?

The run chart in Figure 7.11 (case 1) shows one possible scenario that could have yielded the results observed in the test. The run chart shows results for cycle times for weeks 1 to 14 (three weeks before the change was made until three weeks after the second test observation was made). The run chart in case 1 confirms the conclusion that the change did result in a meaningful improvement.

Figure 7.12 shows five run charts for other possible scenarios that offer alternative explanations of the test results. In each case, a run chart of cycle time for weeks 1 to 14 is shown. The test results for week 4 (cycle time of 8) and week 11 (cycle time of 3) *are the same* for all cases.

> The Friday lunch meeting began with a discussion of run charts. Kerri observed, "Bob, I see many PowerPoint slide presentations with graphics that display two bars, one marked "before" and the other marked "after," with the implication that an improvement has been made [see Figure 7.10]. I am sure you have seen these charts." Bob agreed the bar charts were widely used in the organization. Bob then asked, "Kerri, what has this got to with our topic on run charts?" Kerri then began to build on this chart in order to see data over time—this time on simple run charts.

In case 2 there is no obvious improvement after the change is made. The measures made during the test are typical results from a process that has a lot of week-to-week variation. The conclusion from analysis

Figure 7.11   Run Chart for Case 1

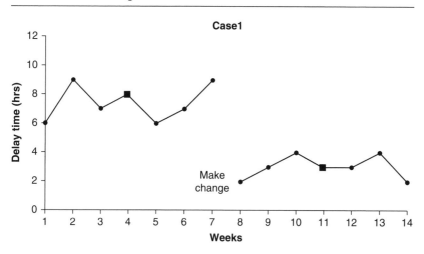

Figure 7.12 Run Charts for Cases 2–6

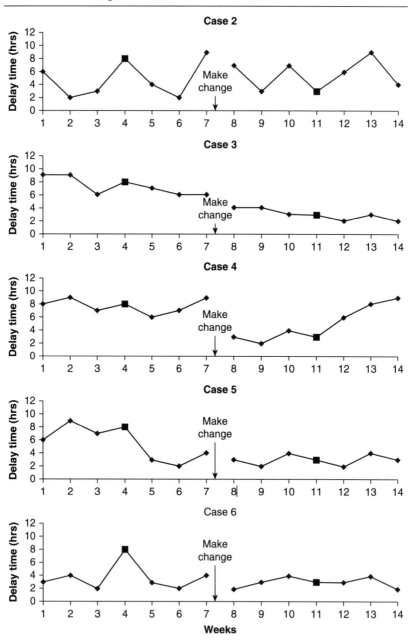

of the run chart is that the change did not have any obvious impact on the cycle time.

In case 3 it appears that the process has been steadily improving over the fourteen-week period. The rate of improvement did not rise when the change was introduced. Although the cycle time for the process has certainly improved, there is no evidence that the change made any contribution to the steady improvement in the process over the fourteen weeks.

In case 4 an initial improvement is observed after the change is made, but in the last three weeks the process seems to have returned to its prechange level of cycle time. The results may be due to a Hawthorne effect. This is named after some tests on productivity conducted at the Western Electric Hawthorne plant in the 1920s. During the test, the people involved may be more careful or diligent in their work, and this extra diligence, rather than the change being tested, may be the real cause of the improvement.

In case 5, an improvement in the process cycle times has occurred, but it appears that the improvement occurred in week 5, before the change was made after week 7. The improvement in cycle time should be attributed to some other phenomenon, not to the change made.

In case 6 the process appears to be stable, except for a special cause that occurred in week 4 when the pretest results were obtained. The unusually high result on week 4 made it appear that the typical result on week 11 was an improvement. Once again, there is no evidence that the change contributed to any improvement.

> "Kerri, I can really see the power of the run charts over time. Since we don't have control limits we could use a test of significance to answer our question on the effectiveness of change. Is this correct?" Kerri responded, "Bob, let's look at the run charts on cases we have here and apply the t-test for significance. I will calculate the p values for you."

If a statistical test of significance (for example a t-test, described in books on statistical methods) for difference in means was used, would there be significant results in cases 2 through 6 in Figure 7.12?

In performing a t-test on the fourteen points of data from each of the cases, case 3 was significant with a p value = .001, case 4 was significant with a p value = .034, and case 5 was significant with a p value = .030. That is, using a statistical test of significance would lead to an incorrect decision for three of the six cases because significance does not prove causality.

"Bob, what are you learning about run charts and our tests of significance?" "Kerri, it is apparent to me that looking at data over time is very important before considering any p value. We would have made some bad decisions here without analyzing the run charts. Many of my colleagues have been taught just to look at the p value and ask no more questions. If the p value is <.05 it is significant. If it is >.05 then ignore the change."

We have discussed the power of simple run charts; earlier we discussed the more powerful control charts. Shewhart developed the control chart method for determining whether variation in a system is dominated by common or special causes. Although there are many situations in which the statistical formality of control charts is useful, often it is adequate to rely on run charts, or simple plots over time.

Leaders should understand the different ways that variation is viewed and be able to explain changes in terms of *common causes* and *special causes*. They should be able to use and insist on seeing data for they have to make decisions in graphical form. Graphical methods are generally easy for everyone to learn and participate in discussions that are important to the organization. Graphical methods have proven useful in speeding up the time to make decisions and take action. Leaders should understand the concept of stable and unstable processes and the potential losses due to tampering. The capability of a process or system should be understood before investing in changes. The theory of variation will be useful to you as you develop and use the components of strategic intelligence.

In their final meeting, Bob informed Kerri that he had met with the leadership team and had shared his learning. "Kerri, the CEO and staff want to learn more and were wondering if you could spend some time helping them understand variation." Kerri replied, "Good for you, Bob, this is beyond my wildest expectations. I would be happy to make a presentation!"

Leadership to Improve Population Health

The use of data to make decisions has a long history. Let's consider one of the historical giants in health care and her use of data, Florence Nightingale.[5]

FLORENCE NIGHTINGALE: THE LADY WITH THE STATS

Florence Nightingale (1820–1910) provides an outstanding example of health care leadership. Nightingale's effective use of data and statistics can be found in her work to improve health care. Her popular public image is *The Lady with the Lamp* tirelessly working to ease the suffering of sick and wounded solders. Less known is her understanding of statistical methods and her ability to present data effectively to gain followers, promote action, and improve the delivery of health care. This ability justifies a different title for Nightingale: *The Lady with the Stats.* Her achievements after becoming famous as a caring nurse are her greatest contributions to health care.

Florence Nightingale lived at a time when western Europeans were starting to make war on an industrial scale. European countries fielded armies with hundreds of thousands of soldiers during the Napoleonic Wars. The Crimean War was the first significant war fought by the British after Waterloo. British battlefield casualties were heavy, but more soldiers died from infection, cholera, spoiled food, bad water, and sanitation than were killed in battle.

One of the worst contributors to deaths from causes other than the battlefield was the Scutari Hospital near Istanbul, Turkey. Florence Nightingale and her team of thirty-eight nurses arrived at Scutari Hospital in November 1854. Although Nightingale's focus was on direct patient care to alleviate the pain and suffering of British soldiers, with her team of nurses she reorganized the hospital, started cleaning it, and convinced the army bureaucracy to provide needed supplies. But the death rate continued to rise. Nightingale's improvements at this time can be grouped into two major categories:

1. Quality of food and water (and nutrition in general)
2. Sanitary conditions and cleanliness

As the mortality rate continued to rise, Prime Minister Palmerston's government sent a sanitary commission to Scutari Hospital in March 1855, six months after Nightingale and her team arrived. The sanitary commission improved ventilation and flushed out the sewers. With these changes the mortality rate, which had begun to level off, began to steeply decline (the run chart in Figure 7.14 is annotated with these changes of the commission and shows the reduction in mortality rate).

When Nightingale returned to England, she was honored as champion for the health and welfare of the average soldier. However, she was haunted by the realization that she had not done enough to save the soldiers under her care. Asked to write a report on her experiences in the Crimean War by Queen Victoria, she spent two years compiling her report to the British Secretary of State for War in 1858: *Notes on Matters Affecting the Health, Efficiency, and Hospital Administration, Founded Chiefly on the Experience of the Late War.*

This report describes Nightingale's use of data to illustrate changes. The report described the improvement of food preservation, cleanliness/sanitation, and the impact of these changes on Scutari Hospital mortality rates. Her report stimulated the army to improve its hospitals. Nightingale's effective and innovative visual display of data are supplemented by use of a run chart to illustrate this technique for testing and evaluating change (the run chart is based on Nightingale's data and some of the statistical methods described in this chapter).

Figure 7.13 shows the number of deaths that occurred from preventable diseases (blue), those that were the results of wounds (red), and those due to other causes (black). Nightingale did not invent this type of chart, but she improved the concept significantly. It resembles a pie chart cut into twelve equal angles that advance in a clockwise direction. Each shows what happened during one month of a year. Each slice describes the deaths that occurred in that month. At a glance, one can see the impact of disease, wounds in battle, and other causes of deaths. Starting with graph 1 on the right, you can see the size of the preventable diseases decrease in graph 2 on the left.

Figure 7.13   Nightingale's Causes of Death Chart

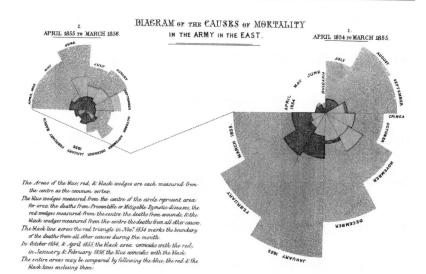

Notice that each slice has three sections: one for deaths from wounds in battle, one for disease, and one for other causes. Battle deaths are small in comparison in every month except September 1855. It was during that month that the last assaults took place at Sevastopol, ending the siege and winding down the Crimean War. By comparison, even the combat that included the famous Charge of the Light Brigade in October 1854 did not result in more deaths than did disease and other causes.

To see this effect using a simple run chart as described in Figure 7.9, see Figure 7.14. Nightingale's information about changes made and their effect are shown on the chart at the time they were predicted to become effective (that is, how long it would take for the effect to show up in data compiled and plotted on a monthly basis).

The effects of the changes are apparent in the simple run chart. After collecting the evidence and constructing the charts, Nightingale came to a difficult conclusion; Bostridge (2011) reports that "Nightingale changed her mind, reaching the painful conclusion that most of the soldiers at her hospital had been killed by bad sanitation, due to her ignorance. She had helped them to die in cleaner surroundings and greater comfort, but she had not saved their lives."[6] More had to be done to protect her boys in the future.

Figure 7.14   Run Chart of Nightingale's Data

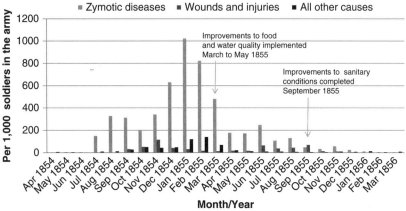

Nightingale Run Chart of Stratified Data
British Army Casualities April 1854–March 1856

She had the moral courage to admit her errors and move beyond regret to take action as a leader for public health. She used her skills with data to gain followers for the cause of improving army hospitals and eventually hospitals throughout the Empire. Nightingale's data and charts helped leaders in the British Army make decisions relative to field practices, which had a significant impact on hospital administration of all types. Once leaders in the British Army saw from Nightingale's chart that cholera, typhus, and dysentery were far more effective in killing British soldiers than were the Russians, they realized that a better approach was needed at army hospitals. This knowledge and her statistically based approach became the foundation of her curricula at the Nightingale Training School at St. Thomas' Hospital in London, which she founded in 1860.[7]

Nightingale's concluding remarks in her *Notes* are forerunner to the concept of differences between enumerative and analytic studies in statistics as introduced, developed, and advanced by the work of Walter Shewhart and W. Edwards Deming: What can we learn from the data to make changes for a better future? Nightingale's remarks:

> The main end of statistics should not be to inform the Government as to how many men have died, but to enable immediate steps to be taken to prevent the extension of disease and mortality.

> It is therefore of paramount importance to have special reporting for special occasions: e.g. the Yellow Fever breaks out in consequence of

the locality or overcrowding of a Barrack, or dysentery in consequence of monotony of diet.

If the government had known, week-by-week, that Scorbutus was ravaging the Army in the Crimea, the very first appearance of the disease in the weekly states with a reason why the disease had appeared at all, would have led the Government immediately to have sought for the requisite supplies to arrest it.

If the Medical Officer waits till the time of reporting comes round, all that is accomplished is that the Government know that they have lost a certain number of hundreds of men in a way which might have been prevented. . . .

Nightingale's insight into the use of statistical methods, not only to summarize and make predictions about conditions, but also to lead to action on the "cause system," was clearly ahead of her time and is a guide to health care leadership to this day.

SUMMARY

- Statistical thinking for leaders contributes to the leader's effectiveness in using data.
- Understanding the difference between special and common cause variation helps the leader minimize the cost of the two kinds of mistakes, overreacting and underreacting.
- Using the five simple patterns of special causes can assist the leader in application of strategic intelligence and asking important questions.
- Graphical display of data is very important for learning. Being able to see data over time helps the leader to explain the effectiveness of changes as they implement their vision.
- If the leader is using a dashboard, simple graphical methods such as the run chart and control chart will clarify the meaning of data. If traffic signals are used, red lights should be reserved for special cause patterns whether they are good or bad news.
- Run charts are simple and effective tools for helping people to understand data over time and the effectiveness of changes.

KEY TERMS

Common cause

Control chart

Control limits

Dashboard

Mistake 1—Type 1 Error

Mistake 2—Type 2 Error

Rules to identify special causes

Predictable

Run chart

Special cause

Stable system

Statistical control

Unstable system

EXERCISES

Study the following case study example[8] and answer the following questions:

- What is the issue concerning variation? Precisely state what measure is varying.
- How is the variation being treated—as variation resulting from common or special cause variation? If special, by what criteria is "special" determined?
- Explain why the correct interpretation of the cause of variation might be switched (common instead of special or special instead of common). What information in the case supports this different interpretation?
- What would you have said or done to help the thinking about variation if you had been present as the case developed?

EXAMPLE OF CASE STUDY

I complained to the postmaster in Washington about mistakes in mail that came to my address. Everyone in the neighborhood, including me, it seemed, received envelopes addressed to other people. As I redelivered an envelope to an address not far away, I was met at the door by a woman just on her way out with an envelope in her hand addressed to me. An even trade. My complaint to the postmaster brought the following reply:

> Mistakes like the one you point out are a source of irritation to us in the postal system, as they must be to you. This problem has been going on for years. We assure that every mistake like the one that you mentioned is brought to the attention of the carrier at fault.

Answers to the Previous Four Questions:

1. The variation issue is that some letters go to the correct address while others go to the wrong address.
2. The variation is being treated as due to a special cause. The carrier that delivers a letter that results in a complaint is treated special ("brought to the attention of the carrier at fault").
3. There are clues in the case that indicate that the problem may be due to common causes:
   a. "Going on for years" indicates this is not an isolated event or a problem that recently started.
   b. "Everyone in the neighborhood" indicates not a localized issue.
4. To help the thinking in this case, first raise the question, "What evidence do we have that any carriers are at fault?" This should result in data collection. Initially, the complaints could be analyzed to see if the problem is a system problem. Then focus on fundamental changes to the system to reduce the common causes that create the possibility of mistakes.

Opportunities for Learning from Variation

1. The supervisor of nurses for the hospital was very interested in making certain that the nurses who posted information to the patient records did them right the first time. To help accomplish her goal of Six Sigma (3.4 PPM Defects), the supervisor sampled a total of sixty patient files from each of the ten nurses during the month and checked them for accuracy. At the end of the month the supervisor met with the nurses who produced more than the average number of errors. She explained the importance of doing the patient records right the first time and asked them to agree to improve the next month.

2. In order to motivate the health care staff to improve patient access, the managing director of a large primary care system established a quarterly patient access goal for each clinic in the system. The clinic managers used this goal to establish individual goals for each of the of the clinician groups in his hospital. Those clinicians that did not meet goals were asked to explain the reasons for the missed goals.

3. A hospital historically had a poor safety record. One step to improve safety that was initiated by the CEO was to rank the hospital departments in terms of the number of patient safety incidents they had over the last three years. The CEO then scheduled individual meetings with those departments who were in the bottom 5 percent in terms of patient safety. During the interviews he urged the health care staff to be safety conscious and stop performing unsafe acts on the job.

4. The accounting group of a managed care organization was responsible for closing the books at the end of each month and providing management with a profit and loss statement for the month. As part of their efforts to increase productivity and cut costs, they established a goal of 200 person-hours maximum to accomplish this task. They believed the goal was achievable, because more than half the months they were able to close the books in less than 200 hours. The method they decided to use to achieve their goal was that for any month in which it took more than 200 hours, a team from the accounting department would analyze the causes of the excess hours. After six months of analysis, suggestions for removing the causes of excess hours would be made to management.

5. Overtime expenditures represented the largest variable cost at the organization's four hospitals. To better control these costs, the regional hospital managers began reviewing the cost reports each month. Explanations and justifications were requested from the hospitals that exceeded 3 percent of their monthly budget for overtime. After one year, deviations of greater than 3 percent had dropped to almost zero, but the total variable costs for the hospitals had increased. In order to better control these costs, a suggestion was made to begin asking for explanations for all costs that exceeded 1 percent of the overtime budget. Another suggestion was to visit the hospital with the largest deviation each month for a budget review.

ENDNOTES

1. This chapter has been adapted from Chapter 4 of *The Improvement Guide: A Practical Approach to Enhancing Organizational Performance* by Gerald J. Langley, Ronald D. Moen, Kevin M. Nolan, Thomas W. Nolan, Clifford L. Norman, and Lloyd P. Provost (San Francisco: Jossey-Bass, 2009).

2. Walter A. Shewhart first published his book *The Economic Control of Manufactured Product* in 1931. This book used the terms *assignable* and *chance cause variation*. W. Edwards Deming noted the change in terms in his book *Out of the Crisis* (Cambridge: MIT Press, 2000): "Shewhart used the term assignable cause of variation where I use the term special cause. I prefer the adjective special for a cause that is specific to some group of workers, or to a particular production worker, or to a specific machine, or to a specific local condition. The word to use is not important; the concept is, and this is one of the great contributions that Dr. Shewhart gave to the world."

3. The presentation of the Hospital Dashboard was adapted from the work of Sandy Murray and Lloyd Provost. This was originally presented at the Institute for Healthcare Improvement's Forum in 2010. The authors highly recommend their book *The Health Care Data Guide: Learning from Data for Improvement* (San Francisco: Jossey-Bass, 2011).

4. The run charts from Figures 7.8 to 7.12 were taken from Gerald J. Langley, Ronald D. Moen, Kevin M. Nolan, Thomas W. Nolan, Clifford L. Norman, and Lloyd P. Provost, *The Improvement Guide: A Practical Approach to Enhancing Organizational Performance*, 2nd ed. (San Francisco: Jossey-Bass, 2009).

5. David Wayne suggested the Florence Nightingale topic and provided a first draft. The authors are indebted for his contribution of the idea and first draft.

6. Mark Bostridge, *Florence Nightingale: The Lady with the Lamp*, http://www.bbc.co.uk/history/british/victorians/nightingale_01.shtml#two, last updated Feb. 17, 2011.

7. It is now called the "Florence Nightingale School of Nursing and Midwifery" and is part of King's College, London.

8. W. E. Deming, *Quality, Productivity, and Competitive Position* (Cambridge: Massachusetts Institute of Technology, 1982), 159.

8

UNDERSTANDING
THE PSYCHOLOGY
OF COLLABORATORS

Adriana Dean, CEO of a hospital system, was having difficulty communicating with people in her organization. She had read several self-help books on better communication, but she felt something was missing. Another CEO told her about his coach, Dr. Michael Maccoby, who had helped him with "personality intelligence" and had given him the tools to better understand his collaborators and partners. Adriana was intrigued and invited Dr. Maccoby for a visit. Before the visit, Dr. Maccoby gave Adriana some pre-work. He asked her to complete two surveys to gain a better understanding of herself and her leadership style. Maccoby explained that they would discuss both during his visit.[1]

In a bureaucracy, people are placed in jobs with defined constraints and measurable outputs. Managers don't need to understand the personalities of employees, just their results. In contrast, a learning organization is collaborative. People partner and interact in teams and on projects. They may propose initiatives and make decisions, individually or jointly.

To work effectively and avoid conflict, they need to understand their own and others' values and motivations.

Leaders will gain willing followers when they are able to fit collaborators into roles that connect with their values and abilities. To be effective leaders and collaborators, people in learning organizations need to develop their **personality intelligence**, their understanding of **values** and motivations that drive behavior at work.

Understanding the people you lead involves awareness of their strengths, motivations, and emotions. It involves learning concepts that sensitize you to patterns of behavior and opening yourself to emotional attitudes. Understanding people requires developing both head and heart.

The concepts you will find useful to understanding people describe intellectual, temperamental, and motivational differences. The *Oxford English Dictionary* (OED) defines *intelligence* as understanding. The psychologist Robert Sternberg studied three independent types of intelligence:

- *Analytic,* the type tested on IQ tests which measure memory and logical ability
- *Practical,* including awareness of people's motives, skill at timing, and tact
- *Creative,* including imagination, pattern recognition, and systems thinking[2]

Although intelligence is partly inherited, it can be developed by study and practice. Clearly, all health care professionals need knowledge of their subject matter and analytical intelligence. However, effective leaders also demonstrate practical intelligence and work on developing their creative intelligence and wisdom. All these qualities are employed in strategic intelligence.

Maccoby arrived to meet with Adriana Dean and discuss the results of the surveys she had completed. First, Adriana reported on her difficulties in communicating her vision to the organization as well as in day-to-day communications. Maccoby then began to discuss personality intelligence and its importance for effective leadership and communication.

Personality Intelligence

A key part of practical intelligence for leaders is **personality intelligence** because it is essential for effective partnering and motivating. Personality intelligence includes both concepts and emotional understanding, both head and heart. The concepts include

- *Talents and temperament:* what we are uniquely born with
- *Social character:* how we are like others brought up in the same culture
- *Drives:* how we are like all people
- *Motivational type:* how we are like some people within our culture
- *Identity and philosophy:* how we are like no one else

Talents and Temperament

Psychological research also indicates that there are five temperamental traits that appear to be genetically determined, but which, at least to some degree, can be strengthened. These, called "**The Big Five**," are

- *Openness* to experience and curiosity, versus just following the same routine. This trait is the motor of continual learning in a world that is constantly changing, and it can be strengthened by practice.
- *Agreeableness* versus suspiciousness. The most effective leaders are trusted in part because they trust others unless that trust is betrayed. Then they have the practical intelligence to cut relationships with those who prove to be untrustworthy.
- *Emotional stability* versus emotional instability. This is a trait that protects a person from being overwhelmed by inevitable setbacks. It is related to resilience.
- *Conscientiousness,* determination, sticking with a task, versus being easily distracted. This trait is essential for professionals and especially leaders who deal with constant demands and distractions.
- **Extraversion,** versus **introversion,** does not predict success or failure. There are effective leaders with each of these traits. However, network leaders tend to be extroverts, and strategists tend to be introverts.

Temperamental traits determine how people behave, not why they behave as they do. The purpose of a person's behavior is rooted in both conscious reasoning and unconscious **drives**, both interests and values. Those interests are often based on a person's sense of identity.

Social Character

Psychological research shows that we are also born with many dynamic tendencies, motivational systems, or drives that, through the socialization process, are shaped into our needs and values. The configuration of drives and values is the human equivalent of animal instinct. It provides a spontaneous way of reacting and adapting to our environment. It becomes a key part of our personality, including those value-drives that are shared by people raised in the same culture, that is, the **social character** which adapts people to survive economically and emotionally in that culture. Our system of value-drives energizes and places demands and curbs on our intellect and identity, which, in turn, can work to shape these values.

Both social character and personality types express the combination of the behavioral tendencies or value-drives that all human beings share. Maccoby has grouped them into seven categories (see the following section). These value-drives can be observed in all infants. As we grow up, they are shaped into our needs and values by family, school, work, sports, close relationships, and our other experiences. However, in different people, they are shaped into different patterns. Some drives become stronger then others. These patterns are what we call personality types.

Human development means the development of value-drives in a way that makes us stronger, consciously able to direct our behavior productively to determine and satisfy our needs to grow and prosper. It means integrating them into our sense of self and, ideally, our philosophies. Lack of development means that these drives become unproductive; they can become addictive needs which can cripple us so that we are driven by them. Psychopathology means that these drives have been distorted in ways that cripple a person. Rather than consciously shaping the self, pathological drives destroy an individual's freedom.

Humans survived early on by inclusion in the group and some societies around the world are still on the tribal side of social character. Some leaders can push an organizational culture into tribalism. The best leaders encourage collaboration, learning, and individuation. They support people who think for themselves and express moral and ethical concerns. Note the word *individuation*. This is not the same as being an individual. Maccoby defines individuation as: *developing one's personality,*

Figure 8.1   Social Character

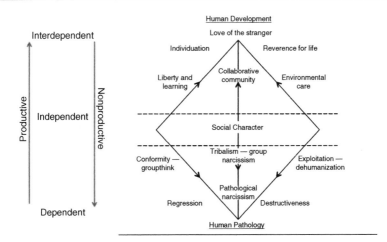

Source: Adapted from Michael Maccoby and Tim Scudder, *Becoming a Leader We Need with Strategic Intelligence.* (Carlsbad, CA: Personal Strengths Publishing, Inc, 2010). Original concept from Erich Fromm, *The Heart of Man* (New York: Harper & Row, 1966), p. 114.

head and heart, so that one becomes able to respond and act according to one's values and convictions about what is right. This is in contrast to conforming to social norms or according to authority, both external and internalized. It means being responsible, able to respond according to one's humanistic conscience.

This diamond (Figure 8.1) was developed by Fromm and Maccoby to represent human development versus human pathology. Few people achieve the ideal of human development that has been expressed in all the great religious traditions including the commandment to love (agapé) the stranger. However, leaders can articulate and practice values that move people in the direction of human development by encouraging collaboration, continuous improvement, learning, individual initiative, and concern for the impact of policies on people and the environment.

Drives

Our drives are in large part shaped by the socialization process—family, school, work, play—and those leaders who structure this process. However, as we grow up, we can become aware of our drives and work to

Figure 8.2   Seven Value-Drives

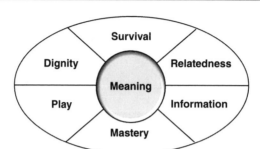

shape them into motivating values by the decisions we make, the habits we form, and the philosophy we construct. Leaders can help to energize followers with inspiring emotions that fire up these values, such as hopes for glory or threats to survival. And leaders can strengthen intrinsic motivation by connecting these drives to a person's role and relationships. Figure 8.2 shows the **seven value-drives**[3] that become our emotionally charged needs and motivating values.

Seven Value-Drives

1. The drive for *survival*. Like all creatures, we are driven to stay alive. However, this drive can be developed, so that we don't just want to protect ourselves but also value and strive to protect others in our family, group, or nation, even at the risk of our own survival. However, this drive can become an addictive need for security, an anxious obsession with threats, real and imagined, that draws energy away from productive activities.

2. The drive for *relatedness*. Babies need to relate to caregivers to survive. Psychologists of attachment theory show that how babies relate to their mothers can shape attitudes to interpersonal relations. However, babies naturally relate to others. As we grow up, we need to relate to others to stay sane; the psychotic is emotionally isolated. As we develop, relatedness becomes caring for others, helping them to develop, and being able to give and receive love. This drive can also become an addictive dependency need.

3. The drive for *information*. Infants seek stimulation, then information. Information determines how we orient ourselves, how we seek pleasure and avoid pain. As we grow up, this becomes a drive

to learn, to gain knowledge and understanding. But this drive can also become an unproductive addiction to information: for example, obsessively surfing the web or scrounging for bits of gossip.

4. The drive for *mastery*. From infancy, we are driven to master our own bodies: walk, talk, handle objects, eat, and so forth. The use of tools and technology increases our brain power. As we grow up, our development includes increasing competence and achievement. This drive can also become an addictive need for control and power over others.

5. The drive to *play*. For the infant, repetitive play is a means of mastery. As we grow up, play becomes an arena of freedom to experiment and innovate. Creative artists and scientists see their work as disciplined play. The spirit of play drives exploration and innovation. When this drive is not developed productively, it can become an addictive need to escape from reality into fantasy.

6. The drive for *dignity*. From infancy, we have a need to feel respected, to experience self-esteem. The frustration of this drive causes shame in early childhood, which can either be a motivation for learning the behavior that a family or culture requires or, if too extreme, can cause crippling humiliation. As we grow up, we are driven to seek **recognition**, honor, and even glory. However, this drive can also become excessive pride, arrogance, or the obsessive need for praise, to feed a lack of self-esteem. An attack on dignity can cause extreme resentment and destructive anger, leading, for example, to murders where the cause is the feeling of being disrespected.

7. The drive for *meaning*. We have the need to make our activity meaningful, so this drive integrates the others. A large part of our identity is the meaning we create for our drives. We seek competence and knowledge to be good craftsmen or professionals, and we want to be respected and recognized for our achievement. The drive for meaning makes other drives into our values, such as security, love, innovation, excellence. We clarify the meaning of our motivations by developing a philosophy of life, and in so doing, we create our unique identities. This philosophy causes us to mediate our drives and values, to set priorities when they are in conflict. However, a compulsive need for meaning can cause us to become superstitious and put irrational meanings on events; our fears or fantasies may cause us to project meanings on to every event.

When Maccoby next met Adriana, he discussed the first personality survey she had completed (Appendix A describes how to access this survey). He told Adriana that based on her answers she was a visionary-exacting type leader. This implied she was motivated to change her environment to fit her vision of improvement, but she also wanted to be sure that changes were sound and could be measured. Adriana agreed that described her and asked about the idea of motivational types of personalities. Where did it come from?

Motivational Types

Freud described three personality types that can be viewed as motivational systems.[4] They can be viewed as patterns of value-drives. In each type, one or more value-drives are dominant and determine the strongest motivational values of that type.

These types, that in many cases are combined into mixed types, are

- *Erotic-loving:* The dominant value-drive is relatedness and the motivational values are caring and helping.
- *Obsessive:* The dominant value-drive is mastery and motivational values are craftsmanship and independence.
- *Narcissistic:* The dominant value-drives combine survival, mastery, and glory (dignity). The dominant motivation is the power to change things and to gain prestige in doing so.

Erich Fromm renamed Freud's types and added a fourth type.[5] He emphasized that each type could be productive or unproductive. The erotic became *receptive*, either productively helpful and caring or unproductively passive and dependent. The obsessive became *hoarding*, either productively hard working and independent or unproductively stingy and controlling. The narcissistic became *exploitative*, either productively entrepreneurial or unproductively manipulative. He called a fourth type *marketing*, and he viewed this type as shaped by the modern service economy, where people are socialized to adapt to continual changes by making themselves into marketable personality packages. The productive type is interactive and flexible, the unproductive is insincere and without backbone.

Building on Fromm, Elias Porter developed a questionnaire that elicited these types or combinations of types.[6] However, he neutralized any negative reaction to the names Fromm used by labeling these motivational systems by colors. The receptive became the Blue altruistic-nurturing type. The hoarding became the Green analytic-autonomizing type. The exploitative became the Red assertive-directing type. And the marketing became the flexible-cohering (a balance of the other types). He called this type the Hub. Porter also showed that the approach we take when we face opposition or conflict may be different from our motivation when things are going well for us.

Figure 8.3 describes the descriptions of the **motivational types** by Freud, Fromm, Maccoby, and Porter. Under Porter, note the combination of types that Porter recognized as "blends" of two types, for example; Red-Blue, or Blue-Green. Porter's use of graphics to plot the motivational

Figure 8.3   Comparison and Summary of Motivation Types from Freud, Fromm, Maccoby, and Porter

Freud	Fromm	Maccoby	Porter
Three normal types, based on earlier explanations of psychopathology.	Four non-productive orientations of adults in society.	Four productive types within a social character, with an emphasis on leadership.	Seven motivational value systems striving for self-worth in relationships.
Erotic	Receptive	Caring	Altruistic-Nurturing (Blue)
Narcissistic	Exploitative	Visionary	Assertive-Directing (Red)
Obsessive	Hoarding	Exacting	Analytic-Autonomizing (Green)
	Marketing	Adaptive	Flexible-Cohering (Hub)
Recognition of blended types	Recognition of blended types	Twelve combinations of above four types based on dominant and secondary types	Assertive-Nurturing (Red-Blue)
			Judicious-Competing (Red-Green)
			Cautious-Supporting (Blue-Green)
Personality differences between going-well state and conflict state are not described.			Two states of personality; independent descriptions of changes in motivation during conflict

types recognizes the complexity of human behavior. Freud, Fromm, and Maccoby also recognized this complexity but Porter took the step to depict it graphically.

Independent of Porter, Maccoby developed a questionnaire to elicit types of leadership styles based on Freud and Fromm. Like Fromm, he describes productive and unproductive aspects of each type but names them by their productive qualities:

- Caring
- Exacting
- Adaptive
- Visionary

> Adriana noted that she did not know much about Freud or his contributions. He seemed like a long-forgotten character. She asked Maccoby to go a little more deeply into Freud's view about personality. Maccoby said, "You might be interested in understanding what Freud meant by the personality as a system." Adriana said she knew a little about systems theory and asked Maccoby to continue.

Freud described personality as a system composed of three parts:

- *Ego:* the mainly conscious part that tries to satisfy human drives
- *Id:* the mainly unconscious sources of the drives
- *Superego:* the conscience, the moral commands programmed in childhood, which can threaten us with guilt if we express impulses that conflict with its commands.

Maccoby has modified Freud and describes the personality system in these terms:

- *Ego:* essentially the same as Freud's definition
- *Identity and values:* composed both of partly unconscious moral commands programmed by parents in childhood (superego) and conscious ideals and values which sometimes conflict with the drives and needs
- *Drives:* largely unconscious, but shaped into values and the social character

Adriana then asked Maccoby to describe the relationships between these ideas. Maccoby approached the white board in Adriana's office and began to draw a picture of how these ideas fit together to explain the personality as a system.

Figure 8.4 describes Maccoby's depiction of these relationships in his personality system.

Figure 8.4   Maccoby's Personality Viewed as a System

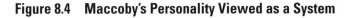

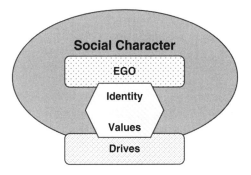

During the discussion of personality as a system, Adriana reflected on her relationship with parents when she was growing up. She said she was the oldest child in a family of three with two younger brothers. Her father was a physicist and her mother a homemaker. She decided early in life that she did not want to be like her mother. She admired her father but she could not identify with him, because she was not a man. She decided she had to develop her own identity and she wanted to change the world to make it a better place. Maccoby and Adriana discussed her development relative to how she answered the survey. Maccoby then emphasized that leaders need to understand their own personalities, including their identities and philosophy of life, before they can understand the people they lead.

Identities and Philosophy

There are two meanings of **identity**; one refers to with whom and for what we identify. This can be the easy answer to the question "Who are you?" In a health care organization, identity as a professional—physician, nurse, manager—may determine a person's interests. Or a person's identity as an African American, Hispanic, union member, gay, or lesbian may be the basis for pursuing common interests. But this meaning doesn't describe a person's values rooted in a motivational system.

The second meaning of identity is the sense of self that integrates personality and gives meaning to motivations. It is who we decide to be and the values we affirm that becomes our personal philosophy. We'll return to this after we have examined the types of motivational systems that make up our personalities.

Effective leaders recognize the importance of creating a **shared identity** for people in their organizations. People identify with and are proud to work in great health care organizations like Mayo, Cleveland Clinic, Geisinger, and Intermountain. Creating a strong shared identity requires that a leader not only communicate a philosophy with a purpose that inspires people, but that the leader also describes and practices the values essential to achieve that purpose. These values, such as quality care, efficiency, and collaboration, will connect with the values of people in the organization. To understand this connection, we need to study how people develop the value-drives that motivate them.

As they discussed personality intelligence, Adriana shared her frustration concerning two types of people she was leading. One type wanted to be told exactly what to do and were great rule followers. The other type seemed to have little or no regard for people in authority but worked well with their colleagues. Maccoby said, "You are describing the two types of social character found in organizations, the bureaucratics and the interactives. Understanding these different social character types will help you craft messages that appeal to both types and to create shared meaning for the organization. Let's talk some more about social character and people with bureaucratic or interactive values."

Bureaucratic and Interactive Values

Maccoby and Scudder have integrated the Maccoby and Porter types in a workbook for a leadership workshop called *Developing the Leaders We Need with Strategic Intelligence.*[7] They also use a questionnaire Maccoby developed to elicit the social character context of these personality types. Maccoby has described two social characters that coexist in organizations at this time: the **bureaucratic** and the **interactive**.

Bureaucratic and Interactive

In Freud's day, children were being raised to succeed in a world dominated by hierarchical bureaucracies. A combination of obsessive-exacting and paternalistic qualities characterized successful bureaucratic people. When Fromm proposed the marketing type (Hub), the number of employees in service work was growing rapidly, while the number of employees in industrial work had reached its peak. Today over 80 percent of the workforce works at some form of service and the most value-producing firms, like health care, combine service with knowledge creation.

Many young people are now being raised with an interactive rather than a bureaucratic social character. Their interactive and adaptive qualities are shaped in families where both parents have careers, and authority in the family is shared. At an early age, with their parents away at work, they are sent to day-care centers where they need to develop interactive skills. Interactivity is facilitated by the Internet and social technology. Interactive people understand that continual learning is essential to keep up with continual change in knowledge work. Unlike in the time of Freud and Fromm, they cannot count on secure employment in a constantly changing global economy and must depend on their adaptive ability and supportive networks to find and compete for employment.

Table 8.1 introduces the concepts of *inner-directed* and *other-directed*. Inner-directed means having a strong superego which is the case with obsessive (exacting-Green) types. It does not mean being individuated (defined earlier) or autonomous. Inner-directed people are governed by guilt. Other-directed people are governed by anxiety that they are not doing what is "appropriate" for their significant others. Interactive people become collaborative only if the organization develops the values and processes that reinforce this norm. Otherwise they may

Table 8.1   Bureaucratic and Interactive Social Characters

	Bureaucratic	Interactive
Ideals	Stability	Continual improvement
	Hierarchy/autonomy	Networks/independence
	Organizational loyalty	Free agency
	Producing excellence	Creating value
Social Character	Inner-directed	Other-directed
	Identification with parental authority	Identification with peers, siblings
	Precise, methodical, obsessive	Experimental, innovative, marketing
Socioeconomic Base	Market-controlling bureaucracies	Entrepreneurial companies
	Slow-changing technology	New technologies
	National markets	Global markets
	Employment security	Employment uncertainty
	Traditional family	Diverse family structures

be interactive but also self-seeking; for example, exhibiting concern only with promoting their own ends or interests, such as people who use Facebook only to advertise their successes.

The difference between the bureaucratic and interactive social characters is summarized by Table 8.1.

Adriana observed, "Dr. Maccoby, until your visit today, what I had learned about motivation in business school was Maslow's Hierarchy of Needs and the importance of paying attention to people from our study of the Hawthorne Experiments." Maccoby noted, "Adriana, let's discuss these ideas a bit, as there is a lot of misinformation about these concepts."

Motivation: Popular Ideas to Unlearn

The topic of motivation is often taught and discussed in the framework of two popular ideas:

- Maslow's Hierarchy of Needs Theory
- The Hawthorne Effect

In both cases, Maccoby has clarified the weakness of these theories and has shown that they support management myths.

Maslow's Hierarchy of Needs Theory

The **hierarchy of needs** theory was proposed by Abraham Maslow in his 1943 paper, "A Theory of Human Motivation."[8] Maslow's hierarchy of needs is often shown as a pyramid consisting of five levels: the lowest level is associated with physiological needs, while the highest level of achievement is associated with self-actualization. According to Maslow, only when lower needs on the hierarchy are met do individuals move to the next levels to achieve personal growth. Higher-tier needs only motivate when the lower-tier needs have been met. Figure 8.5 describes the five levels proposed by Maslow.

Figure 8.5   Maslow's Hierarchy of Needs

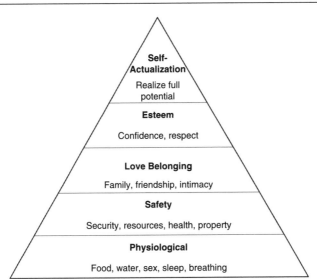

Maccoby's Critique of Maslow's Theory

Maccoby (2007) offered a critique of Maslow's theory. He stated that it is misleading and inadequate as a basis for understanding both individual development and motivation for the following reasons:[9]

1. It doesn't fit the facts of what motivates people at work. It's not based on studies of the values that motivate people, the intrinsic motivation that drives everyone when they have challenging and meaningful work.
2. There is no evidence that by satisfying "lower-level" needs, higher-level needs will automatically emerge. Some people whose needs for money or status have not been satisfied still are motivated to help others or to contribute their ideas at work. People have multiple needs rooted in all seven value-drives.
3. Once personality is formed, needs do not change because they have been met. Empire builders are never satisfied in their need for acclaim, money, and power. However, needs can become more productive. That depends on our awareness, philosophy, and behavior.
4. Maslow's theory of personal development is contradicted not only by everyday experience, but also by neuroscience and cognitive psychology, which show that from birth all of us strive to organize experience, infuse it with meaning, and master our environment. Human development results from opportunity combined with discipline, knowledge, and practice. In contrast to Maslow's theory, we often grow by frustrating rather than satisfying needs.

Maslow's theory may have worked well enough in those industrial bureaucracies where work did not engage the intrinsic motivation of people on the front line. But it doesn't work for a learning organization that needs people at all levels who are motivated to work interactively at continual improvement.

Hawthorne Experiments: Maccoby Critique

When people study organizational development, business management, or leadership, it is not long before they are introduced to the famous Hawthorne Experiments. Starting in 1924 and ending in 1933, a series of studies, led by Elton Mayo and Fritz Roethlisberger of the Harvard Business School, was carried out at the Western Electric Hawthorne factory in Chicago. A stated purpose of the studies was to counteract unions by helping managers gain worker loyalty as well as increase productivity—to make managers more effective leaders. Two main findings on how to lead workers emerged from these studies. One was widely adopted, but the other was misinterpreted and generally ignored for some thirty years because it didn't fit the prevailing managerial context.

The first finding was that workers were motivated not only by money, but also by a caring boss. Mayo, a psychologist and anthropologist, believed that first-line supervisors should get human relations training. The idea, which was subsequently taught in business schools and corporate training courses, was that workers would be motivated to do monotonous jobs if they had a boss who could listen to their problems with empathy. In other words, you didn't have to change the Taylor Scientific Management theory of "one best way." You just had to change the boss's attitude toward workers.

This idea became widely accepted by managers, but it was a management myth. In 1978, when Maccoby asked Jim Olson, then vice chairman of AT&T, why he thought company surveys showed that workers were dissatisfied, he repeated Mayo's teachings: first-line supervisors didn't know how to listen and talk to their people. Olson ignored the fact that AT&T managers had been trying human relations techniques for some thirty years and this had not solved the problem.

The idea that a supervisor should be a kind of psychotherapist was linked in the minds of AT&T managers with their belief in the Hawthorne Effect. However, this was an oversimplified interpretation of the study's findings. This effect was cited to explain a sudden rise in productivity. Supposedly, if you pay attention to workers and experiment with different working conditions, productivity will go up. It hardly matters what you do: you can change their routines, even the lighting in the room, and workers will work harder. Managers at AT&T and many other companies have explained to Maccoby that the **Hawthorne Effect** means that any new workplace experiment will result in short-lived productivity gains that last only until the observers leave and the novelty wears off.

Both of these conclusions were misleading. The workers who were studied at Hawthorne—five women assembling relays (see Figure 8.6)—told the researchers that, yes, the supervisor made a difference, but not because he was an empathic kind of psychotherapist. Richard Gillespie,[10] who studied research notes that were left out of the book, found the following comment about the supervisor: "It was he who injected a spirit of

Figure 8.6   Hawthorne Workers: Women in the Relay Test Room 1930[11]

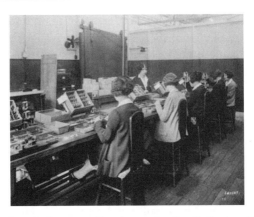

Source: Western Electric Company Hawthorne Studies Collection. Baker Library Historical Collections, Harvard Business School.

play in the group by his comic antics, encouraging them to call everyone by his first name, to take strangers into their facetious conversations, to 'ride' supervisors and fellow operators alike." This isn't psychotherapy, and it's a lot more than paying attention to the workers. It's adding a bit of play to otherwise boring tasks. It's making work fun.

There is also a factor (mentioned by neither Mayo nor Gillespie) that explains why both the therapeutic and playful managers succeeded in motivating the workers: an unconscious transference to a manager who's idealized, even loved, because he's experienced as a good parent.

However, there was another factor that differentiated the therapeutic and playful manager: with the playful leader, productivity increased even more because workers were allowed to decide among themselves how best to do the job. Pay incentives were also a big motivator; productivity rose when workers were paid for the number of pieces they produced. But to admit the efficacy of participation and pay incentives would have undermined the foundations of prevailing thinking that industrial engineers rather than workers could determine the best way to do a job. And it would have ruined Mayo's theory that it was just the caring manager that made the difference.

It took more than thirty years for management training to begin to shake off the message that scientific management plus a caring boss, a combination of hard and soft management, was the best formula for effective industrial-bureaucratic leadership. It took the development of total quality management to show that people responded best when their intrinsic motivation is engaged.

From the discussion about Maslow and the Hawthorne Experiments, Maccoby challenged Adriana to start thinking about how they might tailor this learning for her and her leadership team. Adriana answered, "Dr. Maccoby, I am ready. Let's start thinking about how we put personality intelligence to work!"

Using Personality Intelligence

Understanding social character and personality types can be extremely helpful in motivating, partnering, and avoiding unnecessary conflict. To understand the people you lead, you should first understand your own personality. All of us have the tendency to think that our motivations are normal human nature and we expect others to be motivated in the same way. We are better at recognizing differences in talent and competence than differences in motivational values.

However, you are likely to find a spectrum of types in your organization. Young interactive professionals will resent bureaucratic managers who appear inflexible and overly controlling. Interactive people typically want more responsibility, whereas the bureaucratic people point to the interactive person's lack of experience and view them as having an "entitlement mentality," wanting the responsibilities and rewards without having earned them.

As you lead change, the interactive people will be your allies if they buy into your leadership philosophy. However, professionals with a bureaucratic social character can contribute their knowledge and greater loyalty, if they are motivated to collaborate in achieving the vision.

Creating the Environment for Intrinsic Motivation: The Five Rs of Motivation and the Seven Value-Drives

A learning organization functions best when everyone's intrinsic motivation is engaged. To motivate people so that they become willing collaborators, a leader can employ the **Five Rs**. The Five Rs are *reasons, responsibilities, relationships, recognition*, and *rewards*. People are motivated to support change when the reasons for that change make sense to them. Most people take pride in work that contributes to the well-being of others, expands knowledge, and furthers the common good.

They also want to know how change will affect their responsibilities. Will their new job make good use of their abilities? Will it be meaningful? Will it be challenging and allow some autonomy? People are motivated when their responsibilities are meaningful and engage their abilities and values. The most motivating responsibilities are those that stretch and develop skills and engage a person's values. An intern will be motivated by responsibility for the care of a post-operative patient, but not by responsibility for the complex surgery he has not been trained to perform.

People are also motivated by good relationships with bosses, collaborators, and the people they serve. For many people at work, the relationship with a leader is paramount in determining the productivity of other relationships. A study of employees in the United States reported that the most important factor in having a "good job" was having a good boss. Relationships are strengthened when people are recognized for their contributions. As people work at change, they should have the opportunity to present their accomplishments to the rest of the organization.

Of course, giving out rewards for change, such as bonuses, can strengthen a boss's authority, but it won't motivate knowledge workers to do their work any better, and they may be demotivated by the pressure to conform to a job that is not intrinsically motivating. And to avoid causing resentment that dampens motivation, it is essential that employees consider all pay and rewards to be fair.

Caring (Blue) people are motivated by relationships, especially the opportunity to help people, whereas exacting (Green) types respond to responsibilities that engage their drive for mastery and information and challenge them to use their expertise to improve efficiency. Many of the best physicians combine caring with exacting qualities. They may resist the demand to employ medical pathways where they think that leadership is just trying to cut costs at the expense of the patient's well-being. Only when they are convinced with evidence that the pathways produce measurably better results do they agree to change their treatment methods.

Visionary (Red) professionals want roles that engage a combination of mastery and the extreme of dignity, where they have the power to innovate and receive acclaim.

Adaptive (Hub) professionals, the most interactive type, generally combine one of the other types as a secondary value. For example, an adaptive-helping person will be motivated by being part of a team working together to improve patient care. More than bureaucratic types, the interactive-adaptive people are motivated by reasons. The purpose of their work has to be meaningful to them in terms of its value to others and to their own development. Otherwise, they may be looking around for more meaningful work.

Relationships make a significant difference to all types. The main reason people leave a company is that they don't like their boss or coworkers. They may feel they haven't been respected, recognized for their work, or treated fairly. Caring types respond to warm, supportive relationships. Exacting types want to be empowered to make decisions and recognized for contributions. Adaptive types respond positively to stimulating relationships with colleagues, customers, suppliers, and bosses.

Rewards are extrinsic motivators that can have different meanings to different types. For CEOs, money can be the score they compare with that of their peers. But although money is motivating for piece workers and Wall Street investors, it does not motivate better service from knowledge workers, and some salespeople. In fact, a number of studies show that both primates and humans perform tasks better when they are just solving a puzzle than when they are given bananas or paid for the correct solution. Knowledge workers want to be paid fairly. They can be demotivated if they feel they are being exploited, but they are best motivated by using the other Rs.

For all types, dignity and self-respect depend on being recognized for their work, their *contribution*. Whereas caring types respond especially well to appreciation, exacting professionals prefer the certificates and plaques they can hang on the wall. Visionary people are motivated by the chance to realize their visions. And the adaptive people are motivated by assignments that increase knowledge that beefs up their marketability.

"Dr. Maccoby, I have a confession to make," Adriana said. "I don't think we do a very good job of recognizing the contributions our people make. I think we need to ensure that recognition of real contributions becomes a habit in our organization." Maccoby said, "Regrettably, Adriana, you are probably in a big club. W. Edwards Deming had some choice words about what people want from work. Let's examine something we call the Five Rs and how these relate to the seven value-drives we discussed earlier; these can help build the environment where intrinsic motivation can flourish."

Figure 8.7   The Relation Between the Five Rs and the Seven Value-Drives

---

- **Responsibilities** engages mastery, information, sometimes play, meaning, and dignity (especially with professionals and leaders).
- **Relationships** engages relatedness.
- **Reasons** engages meaning and can engage other drives for different personality types.
- **Rewards** can engage survival, dignity, and meaning. Rewards can combine with recognition as in winning a contest with a prize.
- **Recognition** of a contribution stimulates self-esteem (dignity).

Deming often said that all people want was a chance to have "joy in work." Ron Moen once asked Deming if he thought Michelangelo would have been as productive if he knew that other people would never see his work. Deming implicitly affirmed the importance of recognition and said, "Good question." However, what causes joy or other positive feelings at work are tied to all five Rs.

When leaders can connect work through the Rs to the seven value-drives, the environment can spark intrinsic motivation. Figure 8.7 shows the interrelationships between the Rs and the value-drives.

There are three reasons why recognizing contributions to improvement is not only motivating but also strengthens a learning organization:

1. When the leader of a team is the only person who is recognized for a project's success, those who have contributed feel that their contributions were not so important or appreciated. This is routinely done where improvement experts (for example: black belts, master black belts, and improvement advisers) are recognized but the people essential to their success are not. Make certain that everyone who contributed is publicly recognized when improvements are made.

2. Leaders who take the time to listen to team members as they tell their story, including failed predictions and tests, demonstrate the importance of an organization that appreciates the journey of learning.

3. Examples should be created in the organization from which others can study and learn. These examples can be shared by other organizations inside and outside the health care organization.

What other ways can we recognize teams and individuals who have contributed to significant improvement efforts? The following ideas have been employed in organizations we've worked with.

1. Recognizing people during normal company events or other occasions at which teams and individuals can be recognized
2. Making use of company newsletters, magazines, and other communication tools
3. Sending personal letters signed by a member of top management thanking the individual for contributions to the organization
4. Giving visible tokens of appreciation (books, caps, keychains, and so on)

The Triple Aim—improved health, quality of service, and efficiency—describes reasons that should motivate all personality types, especially when they feel their work makes a difference in furthering the organization's purpose. People want to know the results of their work, and leaders can increase motivation by communicating results and the meaning of results.

The relation between intrinsic and extrinsic motivation is described in Figure 8.8.

People will be motivated when their intrinsic motivation is engaged and they feel they are being treated well and rewarded fairly. They will be resentful if the work is intrinsically motivating but they think their compensation is unfair. If they are paid well, but the work is not intrinsically motivating, they will be compliant, doing the work for the money but with little enthusiasm. And if there is neither intrinsic nor extrinsic motivation, people will be turned off at work, alienated from the organization and its purpose.

A final point about motivation for a learning organization: people will not offer their ideas or accept responsibility willingly, if they are afraid they'll be punished for well-intentioned mistakes. Mistakes should be opportunities for learning. As we have described in previous chapters, they often result from common causes, or

Figure 8.8   Intrinsic and Extrinsic Motivation

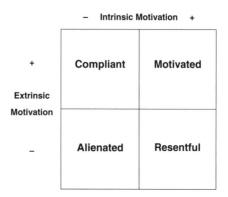

faulty processes. If they are not analyzed but rather punished, the system will not be improved.

Adriana said that she had read a book about emotional intelligence that seemed to have some good ideas. "Could you discuss this idea relative to personality intelligence? I think it is important as a leader to have empathy." Maccoby noted, "Good point. Let's discuss emotional intelligence relative to some other skills a leader can develop."

Leading with the Heart

Awareness of motivational patterns and personality types is one part of personality intelligence. It equips a leader to predict behavior and is a significant aid in selecting partners and connecting to intrinsic motivation. However, recognizing these patterns does not equip a leader to recognize emotions that can influence the behavior of followers, such as fear, anxiety, doubt, resentment, and anger. Effective leaders sense emotions and respond, turning fear into hope, doubt into determination. They are aware when followers feel debilitating anxiety, and they dissolve it by focusing energies on implementing the organizational vision.

They do not paper over anger or resentment but explore and deal with the causes of these destructive emotions.

This part of personality intelligence includes emotional intelligence, but it is better termed "a heart that listens." Emotional intelligence is about self-control and empathy, but personality intelligence goes beyond that to understanding the emotions that people experience in the context of the values that drive behavior. This is the basis for *emotional competency*, the ability to sense negative emotions and then stimulate positive feelings.

Traditional spiritual and philosophical writers used the metaphor of the heart to describe thinking that integrates feeling with logic. The head alone is good for mathematics, science, and crafts, but without a developed heart, one is never sure of what is true in human affairs. Recent neuroscience provides support for this, showing that when the brain is cut off from centers of emotion, people can still do analysis but lose the ability to reason and make judgments.[12]

To develop your heart, recognize that both figuratively as well as literally the heart is a muscle. Without exercise, it won't get strong. Overly protected, it's easily hurt. There's a term for a person with a weak heart and a strong sense of guilt: a bleeding heart, typically someone who doesn't understand others but wants to help the underdog. When the object of these good intentions isn't grateful, the bleeding heart feels taken in. There is also a term for a person who has silenced the listening heart, a hard-hearted person. Hard-hearted leaders rule by fear.

All personality types can develop their hearts, but there are typical differences in attitudes to fully experiencing self and others. To avoid feeling vulnerable or being misled by their emotions, some managers build a shell around their hearts. For example, one such CEO said, "If I opened myself up to people, they would eat me alive." Another said, "I've a shell around my heart, and even my children feel and resent it." But the lack of personality intelligence caused by an overprotected heart cramped their effectiveness. It made these two executives vulnerable to inadequate subordinates who flattered them. This self-protectiveness leaves the unexercised heart flabby and causes managers to obsess over choices when they need to be decisive. The exercised heart becomes stronger through understanding the feelings and values of other people. This results in the ability to make better moral and practical judgments.

In contrast, some managers tend to be more detached. It's easier for them to break off unsatisfying relationships, but it's also harder to commit themselves to others. Although they may have radar-like interpersonal intelligence, they use their gut rather than their hearts in deciding about people. This leads to valuing people too much on appearance, on whether or not they look good, present themselves well, or seem confident. Underneath these quick judgments often lurks unresolved doubt. These types know who's on their side only as long as they're playing the game together.

Of course, some people don't just protect a tender heart, but harden their hearts in the pursuit of power, revenge, or an ideology that justifies terrorism. These are the most dangerous leaders, who are not moved by others' feelings. An example is Fidel Castro, who was remorseless and unforgiving of his perceived enemies and wrote from prison, "I have a heart of steel."

Developing the heart means exercising it, being willing to experience strong and painful feelings; it means that leaders should not ignore the guilt they may feel when making an unpopular decision, firing people, or otherwise causing grief in order to further the common good, and not ignore the anger of those who are hurt. No muscle gets strengthened without painful exercise.

Just as there are disciplines to develop the intellect, such as mathematics, logic, and scientific methods, there are disciplines to develop the heart. They are *clearing the mind* to see things as they are, *deep listening* to get in touch with ourselves, and *listening and responding to others*.

Maccoby related a story to Adriana from one of his colleagues. "Adriana, when my colleague was a teenager his father observed that his listening skills needed to be improved. The boy's father said, 'Son, you were given two ears and one mouth so that you could listen twice as much as you talk.' He then went on to say, 'The greatest respect you can pay to another human being is to listen to them.'" Maccoby then said, "From my experience in working with leaders, the best are able to listen with their hearts as well as their ears. The first step in being a good listener is to clear the mind."

Disciplines of the Heart

Clearing the mind means to see things as they are, frustrating the cravings that cloud the mind, avoiding fantasy and all forms of escapism. Heraclitus wrote that when we dream, we are all in different worlds, but when awake, we are in the same reality. Only when we are fully awake do we see things as they are, and many people go through life half-asleep because they repress uncomfortable perceptions and feelings.

To see things as they are, first of all, we have to practice frustrating the fantasies and passions that keep us from being clear-eyed and fully awake. But we can't frustrate irrational passions if we repress them. At an early age, we naturally repress thoughts and impulses that make us feel crazy or could get us into trouble. But the habit of repression can spread, blocking self-awareness.

Seeing Things as They Are—Deep Listening

This requires experiencing what we would feel and think if we weren't defending ourselves from these unpleasant feelings and thoughts. We have within us all the human potentialities and passions, creative and destructive. An essential function of religious and philosophical thinking is to contain and give meaning to what we can experience when we become aware of powerful and troubling repressed feelings.

But although there's a limit to how much we can simultaneously function in the rough-and-tumble world and explore the depths of our psyches, we can practice getting in touch with what we really experience with other people and not repress uncomfortable thoughts and feelings. Of course, sometimes it's inconvenient to admit to ourselves what we really feel about people we need to get along with. But we can't do anything about improving bad relationships if we don't see people as they are.

There are forms of meditation and prayer in different religious and philosophical traditions that help to connect us to our feelings and silence the noise that muffles the small voice of truth that is in all of us, but often ignored. Also, by paying attention to our dreams, we sometimes become aware of perceptions of ourselves and others that we've repressed because it is uncomfortable to recognize them.

It helps to have a religious and philosophical belief system that can put into perspective our unpleasant or painful experiences and feelings, strengthening our courage to face our problems and overcome them.

Listening and Responding to Others

Listening and responding to others when we have cleared the mind and are awake frees us from the obsession with self, so we can see others more clearly. This kind of listening is active, reaching out with head and heart to understand what we are hearing. Paradoxically, obsessing about what others think of us feeds egocentrism. That just keeps us in ourselves. We only overcome egocentrism when we get out of ourselves to see things from another's point of view—which doesn't mean assuming that others feel what we'd feel in their place. Rather, we need to make an effort to understand how others view things through their own lenses, even experiencing directly what they experience, which is an effort of both head and heart. Beyond understanding is courageous service, reaching out to others, responding with intelligence and passion to social needs.

Not only do we strengthen our ability to understand and act by practicing these disciplines, but also, as Albert Schweitzer wrote, only those who have sought and found how to serve well will be truly happy. By realizing a vocation of service, we strengthen our hearts and also attract others who share our goals.

Finally, a fully developed heart is a courageous heart. The origin of the word courage is the Latin *cor* (heart) combined with the French word for knowledge, courage is acting on knowledge of the heart, in contrast to *guts,* which indicates the kind of toughness required to meet a physical challenge. Courage is acting to defend what you know in your heart to be right, even when that means overcoming fear. Samuel Johnson wrote that without courage, other virtues can't be preserved. Winston Churchill agreed, writing: "Courage is rightly esteemed the first of all human qualities ... because it is the quality that guarantees all others."[13]

People will only fully trust leaders who defend their values and demonstrate courage. Such leaders make a huge difference. They communicate a sense of the possible, a sense that together we can achieve our vision.

The next chapter focuses on creating knowledge in a learning organization. You will see that by understanding motivational values you will be equipped to facilitate learning by avoiding the conflict that can result when people view the same data and events through different value lenses.

Adriana was excited about what she had learned. She said, "I'd like to have all the leaders in the hospital take the personality survey. I think it is necessary for our leaders team to begin learning about personality intelligence as a team. May I call on you to help educate our staff?" Dr. Maccoby answered, "Absolutely. This is a big step for the development of your team and you are right to be leading it." Adriana then asked Maccoby, "What else is necessary beyond personality intelligence." Maccoby noted, "There are four principle areas for development of leaders: (1) strategic intelligence; (2) leadership philosophy; (3) profound knowledge, of which personality intelligence is one part; and (4) methods to build the foundation of the learning organization." Adriana then said, "Dr. Maccoby, let's lay out a development plan for our leaders."

SUMMARY

- Personality intelligence is important for leaders to motivate followers and to develop collaborators to achieve the idealized vision of the organization.
- Personality intelligence includes both concepts and emotional understanding, both head and heart. The concepts are
  - *Talents and temperament:* what we are born with
  - *Drives:* how we are like everyone else
  - *Social character:* how we are like others brought up in the same culture
  - *Motivational type:* how we are like some people within our culture
  - *Identity and philosophy:* how we are like no one else

- Leaders need to understand the emerging workforce of the twenty-first century. Popular literature on leadership may be rooted in a bureaucratic paradigm, filled with myths to unlearn. We are seeing a shift to more interactive social character types entering the workforce who are looking to create value, make a contribution, and are not necessarily loyal to the organization. Leaders need to understand the motivation of this group to engage them in their vision.

- People want more than a job in today's workforce. Health care professionals want their contributions to improving care and serving patients and families recognized. Recognition contributes to their dignity as individuals and professionals.
- Leaders who understand the Five Rs—reasons, responsibilities, relationships, rewards, and recognition—and how they connect to the seven value-drives can help people engage their intrinsic motivation and experience fulfilling work.
- Effective leaders have learned the importance of being able to understand the emotions of others; they develop a heart that listens. They develop skills to clear the mind and to be in the moment, to see things as they are and to listen and respond to others.
- Leaders also have the courage of their convictions. From their leadership philosophy they understand the level of ethics and morality that is necessary for them to have followers and collaborators. On a battlefield the leader must show physical courage. In the professional organization, the leader must show the moral courage to do the right thing regardless of their personal well-being. The followers will be watching and learning.

KEY TERMS

The Big Five

Bureaucratic

Disciplines of the heart

Drives

Extraversion

Five Rs

Hawthorne Effect

Hierarchy of needs

Identity

Interactive

Introversion

Motivational types

Personality intelligence

Recognition

Seven value-drives
Shared identity
Social character
Values

EXERCISES

1. Take the personality and social character questionnaires (see Appendix). What do they tell you about your style of leadership? Ask your team members to take the questionnaires and compare results. What are your strengths as leaders? What do you need to improve? How will you start?
2. Which of the Five Rs are important motivators for you? Are you using all Five Rs in your organization? Describe how you are using them and how you could improve your use of them.
3. To fully develop your personality intelligence, you need to develop a listening heart. Practice being fully present, listening to your own feelings and perceptions, and listening to others with both head and heart.

ENDNOTES

1. We have constructed the conversation between Adriana and Dr. Maccoby that runs through this chapter to illustrate how the ideas presented can be applied by leaders. The conversation has been constructed from Maccoby's experiences with leaders he has coached.
2. Robert J. Sternberg, *Beyond IQ: The Triarchic Theory of Intelligence* (Cambridge: Cambridge University Press, 1985). A less academic presentation of his ideas can be found in Robert J. Sternberg, *The Triarchic Mind: A New Theory of Human Intelligence* (New York: Viking Press, 1988).
3. For a full discussion of the value-drives see Michael Maccoby, *Why Work: Motivating The New Workforce*, 2nd ed. (Alexandria, VA: Miles River Press, 1995), 35–63, 261–264.
4. Sigmund Freud, *Libidinal Types* (originally published 1931), from Standard Edition, Vol. 21 (London: The Hogarth Press, 1961), 215–220.

5. Erich Fromm, *Man for Himself: An Inquiry into the Psychology of Ethics* (New York: Rinehart, 1947).
6. E. H. Porter, "On the Development of Relationship Awareness Theory: A Personal Note." *Group Organization Management* 1, no. 3 (1976), 302–309.
7. Michael Maccoby and Tim Scudder, *Developing the Leaders We Need with Strategic Intelligence* (Carlsbad, CA: Personal Strength, 2010).
8. A. H. Maslow, "A Theory of Human Motivation," *Psychological Review*, 50 (1943), 370–396.
9. Michael Maccoby, *The Leaders We Need and What Makes Us Follow* (Cambridge: Harvard Business School Press, 2007), 22–27.
10. Gillespie, Richard. *Manufacturing Knowledge: A History of the Hawthorne Experiments* (Studies in Economic History and Policy: USA in the Twentieth Century) (Cambridge, UK: Cambridge University Press, 1993).
11. Women in the Relay Assembly Test Room, ca. 1930, Western Electric Company Hawthorne Studies Collection, Baker Library Historical Collections, Harvard Business School.
12. Antonio R. Demasio, *Descartes' Error: Emotion, Reason, and the Human Brain* (New York: Penguin Books, 1994).
13. The Churchill Centre and Museum at the Churchill War Rooms, London, http://www.winstonchurchill.org, accessed Feb 7, 2013.

9

A HEALTH CARE LEADER'S ROLE IN BUILDING KNOWLEDGE

Kerri Barnett was asked by Robert Davis, the VP of Human Resources, to help James Lucian, the head nurse, with an improvement team. Jim said, "Kerri, we have begun a major effort to reduce safety incidents in the hospital. We need a methodology that is practical, not just theoretical." Kerri replied, "Good theory and practice are not mutually exclusive! Recently, I read a book called *The Improvement Guide* that discussed a methodology called the **Model for Improvement** that presents a good theoretical basis for learning and is very practical to use." Jim replied, "Let's get started!" Kerri said, "Jim, let's begin by discussing some basic theory that will help you appreciate the power of the Model for Improvement and how learning about our theories in use evolve."[1]

The previous chapters have described how knowledge of systems, varia-tion, and psychology strengthen a leader's strategic intelligence. Creat-ing and leading learning organizations also calls for knowledge of how we learn, both as individuals and organizations. In a time of continual change, it is essential that we be able to question our knowledge and beliefs and make use of new experiences. This requires us to develop our theories and to be open to revising them. Just as any health care provider's treatment is a prediction based on a theory (diagnosis), a health care leader's strategies and visions are based on theories about what improves effectiveness and efficiency in the organization.

How Do Theories Evolve?

Many of our theories have been taught to us in books or classes, like the diagnostic syndromes taught to medical students. Other theories are developed as we experience and observe events. How does a theory evolve? The process of **theory building** in this framework takes place in two stages: **descriptive theory** and **normative theory**. For each of the two stages we have three steps:

1. Observation
2. Categorization
3. Association

Table 9.1 describes and contrasts descriptive and normative theory[2] relative to these three steps.

Table 9.1   Theory Building Table

Stage	Descriptive Theory	Normative Theory
Observation	1. Observe, describe, and measure the phenomena	1. Observe, describe, and measure the phenomena
Categorization	2. Categorize by the attributes of the phenomena under study	2. Categorize the circumstances in which we are actually studying and learning
Association	3. Develop preliminary statements of correlation; if we do X then Y may or may not happen	3. Develop statements of causality; if we do X then Y will happen or not happen given the circumstances

From the table, we can see that descriptive theories explain our observations and allow us to hypothesize some correlation; however our theory is weaker at this stage of evolution. Additional testing and learning may be needed to evolve descriptive theory. Normative theories are stronger and enable us to predict the results we can expect from changing the way things are done given some circumstances. In both of these stages, developing a theory evolves through the iterative steps of learning: observation, categorization, and association.

What are the practices we observe at high-performing emergency departments? Should practices to achieve high performance be categorized by the annual volume of patients? What are the settings that produce the best results? Are there differences for different patients? As patterns begin to emerge in these associations and important categories are identified, we create models of cause and effect. The models (initial descriptive theories) can then be used to develop normative theory that permits us to predict future observations. When the predictions are correct, our theory is confirmed. If a prediction is incorrect, we want to understand why, so that the categorization can be updated, made more precise, or the theory abandoned. Why does this emergency department have good performance but doesn't use some of the practices included in our initial theory? We may discover that we missed the fact that midlevel providers are used in these emergency departments. We can then update our descriptive theory to make it more useful.

At some point in the theory-building process, the statements of theory switch from association (descriptive) to **causation** (normative). A leader can encourage people to develop changes based on the descriptive theory and test the theory under a wide range of conditions. Good theory building demands that we test to discard or revise theories (disconfirm) rather than test to confirm. The serious scientist wants to know: under what circumstances will our theory break down? When a theory predicts correctly, our degree of belief in the robustness of the theory is strengthened. We have predicted that a change will lead to improvement. If the change does not result in an improvement (an anomaly), the anomaly can be resolved by

- Better measurement
- Revising the theory in use with the new learning (updating the categorization with new observations)

James was thinking about what he was learning. He said, "Kerri, from our discussion about descriptive and normative theory building it seems we have to test our theories to the point that we understand under what circumstances the theory in use breaks down. Is that correct?" Kerri replied, "Yes, I know it seems counterintuitive, but we test to find out the limits of our proposed changes. Many people have learned to test just enough to confirm, only to learn later that the change works with some patients and conditions but not others. Since we are working on safety, we need to make sure our changes are good for the patients given a wide range of conditions, such as experience of providers, different wards, and so on."

In a learning organization the presence of an anomaly that does not match our predictions should not be viewed as failure but an opportunity to build a better theory based on the new information. Unfortunately, viewing a failure of a predicted change in this manner is counterintuitive in many organizations. This is not surprising as most of us have been conditioned and rewarded by schools and organizations to provide the one right answer. Regrettably, this can be a barrier to learning. Consider an experience playing the game "20 Questions" with children; "I am thinking of a number between 1 and 50." The first child asked, "Is it less than 25?" Answer: "No." Immediately, there was an outpouring of groans from the other children and the child looked sad. When the answer is correct, the questioner is rewarded and allowed to ask another question. Yet the intent of the game is to deduce the solution from confirming as well as disconfirming information. Whether the answer is yes or no, there is the same amount of information that can be used to discover the answer. In a learning organization, people understand the opportunity of learning from failures. Art Fry from 3M describes how the failure to develop strong glue led to a product that many of us use every day:

> In 1970 Spencer Silver, a chemist at 3M, was trying to develop a strong glue. But his new adhesive was super-weak instead of super-strong. It stuck to objects but could be easily peeled off. No one knew what to do with it, but Silver didn't discard his new glue. What happened after Fry

realized this new adhesive could make a great bookmark? "The next day at work, I prepared some samples of the bookmark. My colleagues started using their bookmark samples as notes and soon were at my desk saying that they were instant addicts and demanding more samples. As the circle of addiction quickly spread within our product development laboratory, I came to the very exciting and satisfying realization that those little, self-attaching notes were a very useful product. We realized that what we had was not just a bookmark, but a new way to communicate or organize information." The Post-it® Note was born.[3]

In normative theory building, categorization of observations is focused on the different circumstances associated with the anomaly. If the theory fails in its predictions, we try to describe the uniqueness of the situation. If the changes tested in some emergency department did not lead to the improvement predicted, we should identify the circumstances, such as inadequate support from clinicians or administrators, and use that to develop our normative theory. By repeating learning cycles, eventually most circumstances for applying the theory can be categorized, making the theory useful for predictions in future situations.

Once people have adopted a theory, it is difficult for them to modify it or let it go. They tend to ignore or reject evidence that contradicts the theory and look for confirming evidence. When their theories don't produce expected results, they tend to blame practice, not the theory behind it. Argyris,[4] who studied this tendency, distinguished single-loop from double-loop learning.

Single-loop learning occurs when the results of our practice don't fit the theory and we interpret this as a need to change or fine-tune our practice. An example would be a health care provider making a diagnosis, and finding that the indicated treatment did not produce the expected result.

Figure 9.1   Single- and Double-Loop Learning

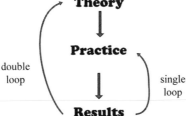

The provider does not question the theory in single-loop learning, but assumes that he or she didn't perform the treatment correctly. With double-loop learning, the provider questions the diagnosis and treatment and is open to new information that can lead to changing them.

> James thought he now understood the concept of single- and double-loop learning. "Kerri, there is an old saying, 'Doing the same thing over again and expecting different results is a sign of insanity.' It also seems like single-loop learning." Kerri replied, "That is pretty good, Jim, and double-loop learning means we have to question assumptions. Sometimes this is difficult; the underlying assumptions may be official policy. To effect a change, we have to gather evidence and present our case to challenge those assumptions."

Some people in your organization will be willing to change their theories and practices when you can show evidence that their theories don't produce the results they expect, or that a different theory leads to practices that produce better results. At a children's hospital in California, some doctors resisted accepting clinical pathways to treat asthma until they were shown evidence that the results of physicians who followed this practice were significantly better than their own. The old saying applies; "In God we trust, all others bring data!"

Learning and Continuous Improvement

People on all levels of an organization may have ideas to improve processes, increase efficiency, or cut costs. In most organizations, they don't communicate their ideas, because they don't believe anyone is listening. Typically, suggestions put into a suggestion box don't lead to results. A lower-level employee opens the box and has to decide about passing the suggestion up the hierarchy. If the suggestion means criticizing someone or changing their practices, it is better not to stir a hornets' nest. The suggestion goes nowhere.

All too often executives are surrounded by courtiers who flatter rather than challenge them. An example: a CEO was presented with survey findings that reported wide distrust of top management by the rest of the organization. He turned to his VPs and said, "This can't be true.

I go around and talk with people all the time, and no one has told me this." The VPs, who knew that no one, including themselves, dared to bring bad news to the CEO, all agreed that there must be something wrong with the survey or the way the questions were phrased.

Furthermore, experts will often resist new knowledge that devalues their experience and expertise, and few experts are willing to learn from anyone other than a certified subject matter expert. Maccoby was once introduced at a meeting of telecom engineers as an expert on leadership, with the implication that anything he said on any other subject should be discounted.

Being open to ideas regardless of their source can lead to improvement innovation. When Maccoby visited a Toyota factory in Nagoya, Japan, a supervisor told him that he had received an average of fifty ideas for improvement per year from each member of his team and 85 percent were implemented. This remarkable result was achieved by instituting a process whereby all ideas were evaluated weekly by a team of supervisors. Ideas might be as simple as improving illumination or expanding a particular job. When ideas were implemented, workers received points which could be used for rewards such as dinner for a couple.

You cannot expect that experts at any level will transform themselves and become respectful to nonexperts and be willing to learn from them, whether they be employees, customers, or patients. To learn from everyone in an organization, you must establish processes for continuous improvement that are integrated with the organizational system and the practical values that further its purpose.

People will also resist change when it challenges their values or interests. They become closed to learning, and they ignore or find reasons to distrust evidence that conflicts with their beliefs. Some physicians at a medical school refused to consider changing their practice to adopt proven pathways, saying that the vice president who was promoting evidence-based medicine was only interested in saving money, not caring for patients. To overcome this resistance, the vice president had to clarify his philosophy, emphasizing that his purpose was both better care and cost savings and that the practical values needed to achieve this purpose included evidence-based practice and continual learning.

Of course, people can also resist knowledge that threatens their interests. Typically, product managers at companies resist learning about and supporting innovations that will draw customers away from their products. IBM had to create a new business for laptop computers located far from the managers of mainframes who felt threatened by the new product and who argued that it had no future. In similar fashion, a Norwegian oil company had to create a new company to protect ships that explored for oil from the managers of the much more costly platforms who saw the ships as a threat to their control of oil exploration.

Fear—whether of losing money, power, status, or of being punished for mistakes—blocks learning. Health care providers learn from morbidity and mortality rounds, but they will resist reporting mistakes and learning from them if they are punished for honest mistakes.

Organizations will learn only if, as Deming emphasized, leaders drive out fear.[5] At AT&T, technicians sometimes cut cables by mistake, resulting in many calls being lost. Because they were afraid of being punished, they didn't report their mistakes. As a result, there was no learning about how to avoid these mistakes or to correct them quickly. Only when a new head of the network instituted a policy of no punishment for reporting mistakes did a design team develop a process for avoiding and correcting cable cuts.

> Kerri was happy with the discussion that she and James were having about the power of theory building. However, she expressed a concern to James: "Jim, when I am working with improvement teams we generally have a difficult time initially obtaining data that is useful to help us with the improvement effort. Generally, what we get in terms of data is the data that is available rather than the data we need for improvement. Usually the first problem we run into is having good **operational definitions** for the data collected." Jim said, "Tell me more." Kerri replied, "What do we mean by a fall? How to we measure length of stay? Just about anything we want to measure usually has an issue with what we mean by the terms we use."

Shared Meaning and Operational Definitions

Organizational learning also depends on shared concepts and a shared philosophy. Operational definitions are necessary to create shared meaning. An operational definition should include

- A method of measurement or test.
- A set of criteria for judgment. For example, suppose the organization is trying to learn how to avoid patient "falls." However, the

simple concept of "falls" can be defined differently. Consider the following definitions of a fall:[6]

- A sudden uncontrolled, unintentional downward displacement of the body to the ground or other object, excluding falls resulting from violent blows or other purposeful actions.
- Inadvertently coming to rest on the ground, floor or other lower level, excluding intentional change in position to rest in furniture, wall, or other objects.

As surprising as it may be, it seems that there is no universally accepted definition of what we mean by a fall in health care. How a fall is defined can be very different from the perspective of the patient or caregivers. The elderly may consider a fall to be the loss of balance. Health care professionals may focus on the consequences of the fall to determine if a fall has occurred. If you are interpreting data from your organization on falls, then the definition becomes important. Have we created a definition that is not sensitive to patients? Has the definition made us blind to an increase in falls? Is the definition so precise that it has overstated the issue and caused an overreaction by our staff, thus wasting resources?

James challenged Kerri. "Kerri, when are we going to get to the Model for Improvement? I am eager to put these ideas to work!" Kerri replied, "Great Jim, you are right on time, that is our next topic!

Utilizing a Standard Methodology for Learning in the Organization

It is important to have a common road map to guide the efforts to improve throughout the organization. The Model for Improvement provides this function. The Model for Improvement contains two basic components:

1. Three questions needed to guide any improvement or change effort
2. The Plan-Do-Study-Act (PDSA) cycle

Given the complexity of the improvement effort one might be able to take all the action necessary by answering the three questions. As a method for improvement, the model becomes a flexible framework for focused questions and, if appropriate, the use of application-specific tools and methodology. It also serves as a guide for building required knowledge and for taking action toward accomplishing desired results. This view leads to a set of questions that form the basis of improvement:

1. What are we trying to accomplish?
2. How will we know that a change is an improvement?
3. What change can we make that will result in improvement?

> Kerri noted, "Jim, if I can answer the three questions and identify a change on the back of an envelope, then I am going to start testing quickly. This provides a quick way to accelerate the rate of improvement. If the challenge is more complex, I find that I can get a good framing with the three questions on one page, which we call the Accelerated Model for Improvement (Ami™) Charter." James exclaimed, "One page! I will believe that when I see it!" (See Chapter 11 for the one-page Ami™ Charter.)

These questions form the basis of a "trial and learning approach." The word "trial" suggests that we are going to test a change. "Learning" implies that we have some criteria by which to evaluate the trial. The focus on the questions accelerates the building of knowledge by emphasizing a framework for learning, the use of data, and the design of effective tests or trials. Before any changes are attempted, learning from testing changes on a small scale is stressed rather than learning from extensive study. Figure 9.2 depicts the Model for Improvement which includes the three basic questions of the PDSA cycle.

The second component is called the PDSA cycle, which has its foundation in the scientific method. The four parts of the PDSA cycle should accomplish the following relative to learning:

- *Plan:* The activity for developing, testing, or implementing changes was planned, including a plan for collecting data for each type of PDSA cycle.

- *Do:* The plan was attempted.
- *Study:* Time was set aside to analyze the data and study results.
- *Act:* Action was based on what was learned.

Kerri said, "Jim, we have discussed the overall Model for Improvement and the use of the three questions. The next part of the Model for Improvement is something we call PDSA." Jim stopped Kerri and asked, "Kerri, when I went to school in the UK and we would take our pet to the vet, it was called the 'People's Dispensary for Sick Animals or PDSA'! I am assuming this is something different?" Kerri laughed and said, "I should have said **PDSA cycle**! Let's revisit our discussion about theory building as we discuss, Plan-Do-Study-Act, not the People's Dispensary for Sick Animals!"

Figure 9.2   The Model for Improvement[7]

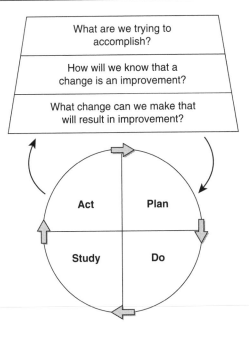

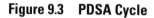

Figure 9.3   PDSA Cycle

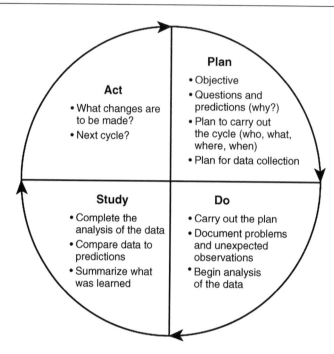

Figure 9.3 describes the four parts of the PDSA cycle.

Richard Feynman, the Nobel physicist, once noted, "Science begins and ends in questions."[8] So does the science of improvement. Being able to articulate the questions to be answered in the PDSA cycle requires some skill. Being able to pose the appropriate questions leads us to improvements that will prove useful in the shortest amount of time. Dennett (2006) has observed:

> Anybody who has ever tackled a truly tough problem knows that one of the most difficult tasks is finding the right questions to ask and the right order to ask them in. You have to figure out not only what you don't know, but what you *need* to know and *don't* need to know, and what you need to know in order to *figure out* what you need to know, and so forth. The form our questions take opens up some avenues and

closes off others, and we don't want to waste time and energy barking up the wrong trees.[9]

Once questions are posed we need to examine our assumptions. We do this by making predictions relative to the questions posed. Prediction requires a theory. We are not guessing. A theory represents our current knowledge about how something in our world works; a process, service, or system. People engaged in an effort to improve should state their predictions by making their *theories in use* (or hypotheses) explicit. Stating theories or assumptions guides in the design of tests to validate or disprove these theories; we can then improve our ideas for change on the basis of the results of the tests. If changes tested do not lead to the improvement predicted, we should identify the circumstances present and use this understanding to further refine our theory. As Einstein once noted, "It only takes a data point of one to cause us to throw out or revise a theory."[10] For example, we may find that changes successfully made in some hospital wards are not successful in others. On investigation, we may theorize this is due to the size of the ward, the lack of support from consulting physicians, or inadequate inpatient capacity in the ward. What changes will be successful under these circumstances? Skillfully building knowledge by making changes and observing or measuring the results is the foundation of improvement.

By repeating learning cycles, we can categorize the circumstances important for applying the theory in the real world, making the theory useful for predictions in future situations. This iterative deductive and inductive approach to learning and improvement is illustrated in Figure 9.4. **Deductive learning** and **inductive learning** are built into Plan-Do-Study-Act (PDSA) cycles. From Plan to Do we use the deductive approach. A theory is tested with the aid of a prediction. In the Do phase, observations are made and any gaps from the prediction are noted. From Do to Study the inductive learning process takes place. Gaps (anomalies) to the prediction are studied and the theory is updated accordingly. Action is then taken on the new learning.

What does this iterative process look like over time? Figure 9.5 describes three improvement efforts that are developing, testing, and implementing changes. From the figure you can see that one team has had the experience of increasing their degree of belief that the changes

Figure 9.4   PDSA, Deductive and Inductive Learning

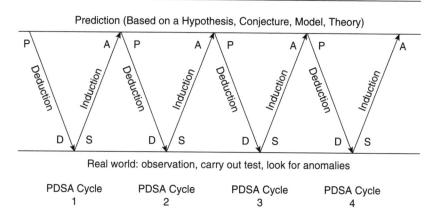

Figure 9.5   Application of the PDSA Cycle to Increase Degree of Belief

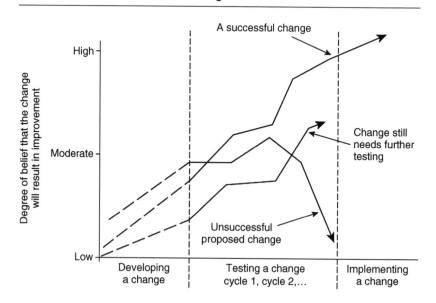

Figure 9.6   Using Multiple PDSA Cycles to Build Knowledge

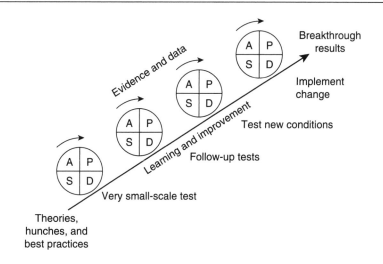

being developed and tested will in fact result in improvement. Another team requires further testing to increase their degree of belief. However one team discovered in testing that their perceived change has proven to be unsuccessful. It is back to the drawing board to develop another change to address the challenge. However, it should be noted that the team has increased knowledge of the subject matter under study even though the degree of belief has plummeted for this particular change. Figure 9.6 describes the increase of knowledge as we move from theories, hunches, and best practice to testing. Even failed tests increase our knowledge.

The Improvement Guide (2009) contains more detailed information on the Model for Improvement and its use. Chapter 10 provides some examples of project charters using the Model for Improvement to establish and lead improvement efforts in a health care setting. These forms and other support materials can be downloaded from www.pkplearn .com (note: permission can be gained through this site to access the forms to support the Model for Improvement).

By testing our theories and using the Model for Improvement, we increase our ability to learn together.

Using Multiple PDSA Cycles to Build Knowledge

Jim said, "Kerri, I can see where PDSA and the iterative use of the cycle depend on our ability to pose good questions. In addition, the PDSA cycle is essential to test our theories and not just to confirm but sometimes disconfirm our beliefs. This seems counterintuitive to what we have been taught in school about the importance of being right and getting the right answer. It seems that the science of improvement expects us to test our theories rigorously to understand where they will break down in practice." Kerri added, "That is correct, Jim. Since we are talking about patient safety, why should we expect anything less than good science?" Jim replied, "Absolutely, let's get that one-page Ami™ Charter out and start charting our improvement journey!"

We learn together when we are able to question each other's theories and beliefs and avoid unproductive conflict. Figure 9.7 describes a way of thinking about developing shared understanding. Consider two people who interpret the same reality differently. They will not gain a common understanding if they attack each other, label each others' ideas, or avoid working at understanding.

In Figure 9.7, there are two ladders labeled "storytelling" that represent how two people process data and experience to arrive at and frame their beliefs. If they do not agree, they should follow the learning rules listed on the figure to avoid unproductive conflict and learn together. These rules call for clearly advocating ideas but providing the data, facts, or reasons that support these ideas. Participants should invite inquiry about how they secured their data and developed their reasoning. Many of our clients have built these learning rules into their team norms so that they are used routinely whether there is disagreement or not.

We can view the same events, behaviors, and data through different lenses. Our personality intelligence should alert us to the different values that sensitize us to different aspects of a situation. For example, a nurse may view a patient's complaints through a caring lens, focusing on alleviating pain, whereas a physician views the same data through an analytic lens focusing on a plan of treatment. The more we understand each other's values, the better we will learn together and avoid conflict.

Figure 9.7 Getting to Shared Meaning, Ladder of Inference, and Learning Norms[11]

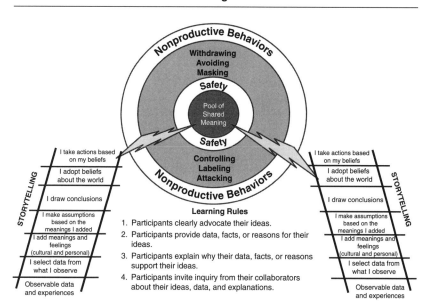

When dealing with conflict or differences, Mary Parker Follett has advised us to assume that both sides are right.[12] As we consider Figure 9.7 and entertain conflict in our own lives, this is probably good advice, especially for a leader who has to be open to different opinions and stories. Using questions to get everyone back to the base data and then to share the journey of learning will reduce the need to be right and more important, the blame-game. In addition, it is important not to become fixated on *what* is right, but remain open to inquiry and learning. The leader should be prepared to be the conductor on this journey on the ladder of inference and to model a behavior of honest inquiry to use conflict and diversity of desires not to compromise but to integrate both interests for a win-win solution. Follett gives the following example of not compromising but developing a new solution that is acceptable to both parties:

> [W]hen two desires are integrated, that means that a solution has been found in which both desires have found a place, that neither side has had to sacrifice anything. Let us take some very simple illustration. In the

Harvard Library one day, in one of the smaller rooms, someone wanted the window open. I wanted it shut. We opened the window in the next room, where no one was sitting. This was not a compromise because there was no curtailing of desire; we both got what we really wanted. For I did not want a closed room, I simply did not want the north wind to blow directly on me; likewise the other occupant did not want that particular window open, he merely wanted more air in the room.[13]

Jim said, "Kerri, I would like you to present to my team and help me with the project." Kerri replied, "No problem, just one promise." James asked, "What do you need from me?" "To help me teach," Kerri replied. "As you teach, you will learn even more!" Jim said, "Say no more—count me in!"

Follett also observed that creating a win-win situation is not always possible; for example, two men that want to marry the same the woman. This will be a win-lose.

Chapter 11 presents additional tools you can use to begin the process of change.

The Leader as Learner and Teacher

The best leaders are passionate learners. When needing to decide about developing a new product or acquiring a company, GE CEO Jack Welch wanted to learn everything he could about the matter. He would take what he called a "deep dive" into the available material. Microsoft CEO Bill Gates took two weeks off each year to study a new area. When he heard of a new surgical technique, William Mayo would go to where it was being practiced and stay there until he had learned it. He would then return home to teach the technique to the surgeons at his clinic.

However, in a complex health care organization, leaders cannot know everything they would like to know to solve problems and make decisions. They need to combine humility with confidence. Humility means that they don't have to know more than anyone else, that they are willing to learn from others. It is also recognition that they may never have all the information needed to make a rational decision. But leaders also need to develop confidence that they can learn enough to make good decisions, and to modify their theories if necessary.

The leader of a learning organization will be a mentor and teacher who motivates others to learn by driving out fear, welcoming new ideas, and instituting processes that facilitate learning. These include open dialogue where no one fears punishment or humiliating put-downs. Also, experiments that test new approaches will be encouraged. Everyone in the organization will learn that all work is a process that includes planning, doing, evaluating or checking, and acting or adapting according to what has been learned. More important, everyone should learn how their work processes and roles contribute to the achievement of the organization's purpose.

The leader will communicate a philosophy with values that determine decisions. But he or she also will be a principled pragmatist who tests these values to make sure they further the organization's purpose and produce the expected results. And if they don't, the values will be modified. In this way, the leader will model the qualities essential for continual individual and organizational learning.

Information in a bureaucracy is supposed to flow upward to the executives who should make decisions. The leader in a bureaucracy is supposed to be the person who has all the answers. In contrast, information in a collaborative knowledge organization is constantly accumulating on the front lines. The challenge for executives is to learn from people who are closest to the customers, patients, and clients. Leaders will not learn unless they are able to ask useful questions and use the learning to help design effective processes.

To develop your theories and improve your knowledge, the following methods have proven useful.

1. Record your predictions.
2. Consider why other outcomes might have occurred.
3. Develop operational definitions of concepts.
4. Ask open-ended questions to confirm or disconfirm your beliefs, not just yes-or-no questions.
5. Use control charts and the theory of variation (see Chapter 7) to understand and interpret key measures. Understanding if the issue is related to special versus common cause variation can lead to very different actions.

6. Test and experiment; usually on a small scale until the degree of belief is such that implementation can be executed with minimal risk of failure.
7. Present data with graphical methods such as run charts, control charts, and Pareto charts.[14] Graphical methods help to involve everyone who has interest in the data being discussed.

SUMMARY

- The importance of theory and how theories evolve from descriptive to normative was discussed. Observation, categorization, and association define how descriptive and normative theories evolve. A useful theory helps us to predict the future. As theories move from descriptive to the normative state they become more useful for prediction.
- Learning from failure is critical to advancing knowledge. Failure is not shunned in organizations where learning and innovation are valued. Leaders help to ensure that it is safe to contribute and learn.
- The distinction between **single- and double-loop learning** is important for leaders to understand. Double-loop learning causes us to question our assumptions and this can be threatening.
- Leaders model learning by both learning and teaching.
- The Model for Improvement provides a robust methodology that employs the PDSA cycle as an engine for learning. The PDSA has the iterative process of deductive and inductive learning that allows us to evolve our theories from the descriptive to the normative, actionable state.

KEY TERMS

Causation

Deductive learning

Descriptive theory

Inductive learning

Model for Improvement

Normative theory

Operational definition

PDSA cycle

Single- and double-loop learning

Theory building

EXERCISES

1. Using the three questions from the Model for Improvement, address a challenge in your organization that needs to be improved:

   - What are we trying to accomplish?
   - How will we know that a change is an improvement?
   - What change can we make that will result in improvement?

2. List three concepts used in your organization every day that might need an operational definition to improve shared meaning. Examples might be: What do we mean by Length of Stay (LOS)? What do we mean by a fall for a patient? Test these definitions with your colleagues; is there shared meaning?

3. Consider using the learning rules from Figure 9.7 to encourage learning in your team.

ENDNOTES

1. We have constructed the conversation between Jim and Kerri that runs through this chapter to illustrate how the ideas presented here can be applied to leaders. The conversation was constructed from our experience with leaders we have coached.

2. Ideas related to descriptive and normative theory were adapted from Paul R. Carlile and Clayton M. Christensen, "Practice and Malpractice in Management Research," Version 6.0 (January 6, 2005). Access to this paper is granted by the author from the book *The Innovator's Solution— Creating and Sustaining Successful Growth* by Clayton Christensen and Michael E. Raynor (Cambridge: Harvard Business School Press, 2003). See Chapter 1 notes, #17, p. 26.

3. "Fascinating facts about the invention of Post-it Notes by Arthur Fry and Spencer Silver in 1974" http://www.ideafinder.com/history/inventions/postit.htm. (accessed November 2012).

4. Chris Argyris, "Double Loop Learning in Organizations," *Harvard Business Review*, September-October (1977), 115–125.

5. Drive out fear, so that everyone may work effectively for the company (see Ch. 3). W. Edwards Deming, *Out of the Crisis* (Cambridge, MA: MIT Press, 2000), p. 24.

6. APS Healthcare, Inc. Southwestern PA, Health Quality Unit, June 2010. Definitions are highlighted from various organizations in Appendix A of this report.

7. Figures 9.3 to 9.6 have been adapted from Gerald J. Langley and others, *The Improvement Guide: A Practical Approach to Enhancing Organizational Performance,* 2nd ed. (San Francisco: Jossey-Bass, 2009).

8. Richard Feynman and Jeffrey Robbins (Ed.), *The Pleasure of Finding Things Out: The Best Short Works of Richard P. Feynman* (Cambridge, MA: Perseus, 1999).

9. Dr. Daniel C. Dennett, *Breaking the Spell: Religion as a Natural Phenomenon* (New York: Viking Press, 2006), 19.

10. This quotation is often attributed to Albert Einstein. His original quote read: "No amount of experimentation can ever prove me right; a single experiment can prove me wrong."

11. Figure 9.7 has been adapted from Kerry Patterson, Joseph Grenny, Ron McMillan, and Al Switzler, *Crucial Conversations Tools for Talking When Stakes Are High,* 2nd ed. (New York: McGraw-Hill, 2011). This work has been combined with contributions from Chris Argyris for the "Ladder of Inference" and "Learning Rules" for groups in Chris Argyris, *On Organizational Learning,* 2nd ed. (Oxford: Blackwell, 1999).

12. Pauline Graham, *Mary Parker Follett—Prophet of Management: A Celebration of Writings from the 1920s* (Washington, D.C.: Beard Books, 2003), 4.

13. Henry C. Metcalf and L. Urwick (1941), *Dynamic Administration—The Collected Papers of Mary Parker Follett* (New York and London: Harper & Brothers, 1941), 32.

14. Pareto analysis is a statistical technique that is used to select the limited number of tasks that produce significant overall effect. It uses the Pareto principle—the idea that by doing 20 percent of work, 80 percent of the advantage of doing the entire job can be generated.

PART 3

Learning from Other Leaders and Creating a Path Forward

THREE CASE STUDIES: MASTERING CHANGE

Health care organizations we've studied and worked with, such as Intermountain Healthcare, Mayo, and Geisinger, have become much admired models for continual improvement and learning. Cliff and Jane Norman have been consultants to the three organizations presented in this chapter, and Jane was temporary chief operating officer (COO) for OCHIN. As they worked with these organizations, they have not only taught methods for developing a learning organization, but they have also learned and expanded their understanding of methods for leaders to build a learning organization (see Figure 10.1). They have been knowledge leaders collaborating with the organizational leaders you'll meet in these cases.[1]

- **A System for Mastering Change in Jönköping County Council (Sweden):** This is an example of how leaders improved patient care, lowered costs and applied their learning to improving community health. Jönköping has also been active in sharing its experience in Sweden and internationally. The Jönköping case will describe how leadership is shared not only in the leadership of the health care organization but throughout the county council.
- **A Medical Leader Improves Care in a Dialysis Clinic:** This case describes the work of Jerry Jackson, MD, to improve care transitions

Figure 10.1 Methods for Leaders to Build a Learning Organization

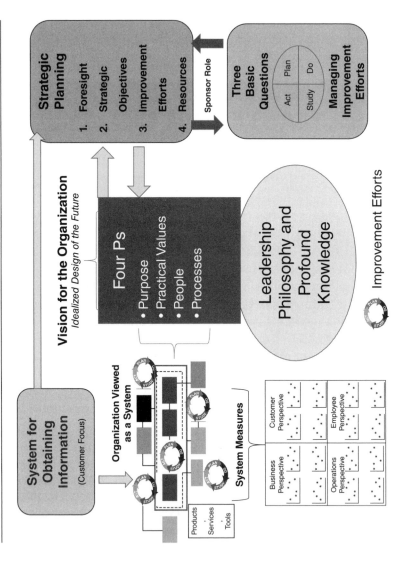

from a hospital to a clinic. Jackson provides a good example of a doctor as leader in developing a learning organization that maintains traditional medical values of patient care.

- **Building a Learning Organization at OCHIN: OCHIN** is a collaborative provider for health records technology, research, and innovative care solutions in thirteen states. They host the largest health care database for the medically underserved within the United States while serving as Oregon's Regional Extension Center. In this role, OCHIN has created a network of health care professionals which share knowledge and solutions working together as catalysts for change and improvement. The case describes how a bureaucracy was transformed into a learning organization.

Each organization began by assessing themselves using the Strategic Intelligence Inventory found in Chapter 11. As these organizations had different strengths within these components, they each approached laying the foundation for their learning organization in a different sequence of events, which is reflected in the flow of each case study. However, each case study will highlight lessons from the book in three categories:

1. Strategic intelligence
2. Profound knowledge
3. Methods for building a learning organization foundation (see Figure 10.1)

The matrix shown in Table 10.1 will allow the reader to identify the methods and tools used within each of the case studies.

Table 10.1   Strategic Intelligence and the Four Ps

Components	Methods	Tools/Concept	Case Study
Purpose and Practical Values	Four Ps	Purpose statement Role description	Jönköping Dialysis OCHIN
Processes: Systems View of the Organization	Macro, meso, micro system mapping	System map (linkage of processes) Role description	Jönköping Dialysis OCHIN

(continued)

Table 10.1 Continued

Components	Methods	Tools/Concept	Case Study
Partnering	Partnering continuum	Commodity supplier Preferred supplier Value-added supplier Strategic partnership	Jönköping Dialysis OCHIN
People	Personality assessment Conflict sequence	Strengths deployment inventories (SDI) Role description	OCHIN
Results: System Measures	Family of measures	Run charts Control charts Role description	Jönköping Dialysis OCHIN
Information Sources: Aid to Foresight	Surveys Best practices Benchmarking	Sources of learning Checklists Use of change packages	Jönköping OCHIN
Visioning: Idealized Design of the Future	Idealized design of the future	Use of the Four Ps	Jönköping OCHIN
Planning to Achieve the Purpose and Implement the Vision	Identifying strategic objectives budgeting resources Identifying improvement efforts	Affinity diagram Driver diagram Priority matrix Gap analysis	Jönköping OCHIN
Managing Change Efforts	Model for improvement	Ami™ Charter team selection grid Charter approval Format sponsor report Format PDSA (Plan-Do-Study-Act)	Dialysis
Management System for Integrating Changes and Improvement	Creating a learning and innovation center	Generic improvement system map	Jönköping Dialysis OCHIN
Motivating and Empowering	Five Rs (reasons, responsibilities, relationships, recognition, rewards)	Role statement Role description document	Jönköping Dialysis OCHIN

CASE STUDY A: SYSTEM FOR MASTERING CHANGE IN JÖNKÖPING COUNTY COUNCIL, SWEDEN

The Challenge

The leadership of the Jönköping County Council is driven by a purpose, vision, and practical values. Key partnerships were developed to create a learning organization. The motivation to implement the vision results from the shared purpose to ensure that patients and families are cared for in the county.

Jönköping County Council is an organization with more than 9,000 employees.[2] On a typical day, 6,100 persons visit the health care services, 1,500 visit specialist physicians, 1,300 visit general practitioners, 300 visit private doctors, approximately 160 are admitted to hospitals for treatment, and 9 children are born.

The **county council** is organized in three health care areas. Each area consists of a hospital with an emergency room and several primary care centers.

This case is not about a number of successful projects; it is about how leaders work to get all the processes in the system working together and show results at the system level. This requires the creation of an organization that learns to achieve desired results and make this effort sustainable. Figure 10.2 describes several measures that have been impacted in a positive direction by the efforts of the Jönköping County Council leadership team.

Figure 10.2   Measures of Performance for Jönköping County Council

Figure 10.2A   Waiting Time

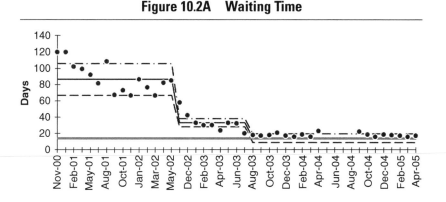

Figure 10.2B   Number of Deaths

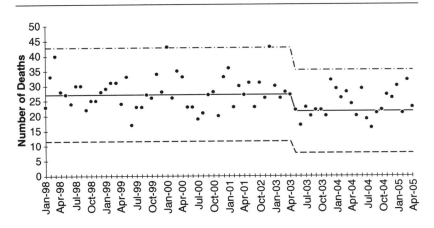

Figure 10.2C   Percent of Operations Versus Visits:
Jönköping, January 2007 to November 2009

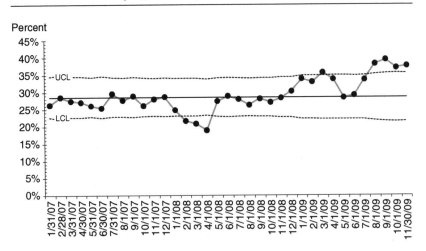

Figure 10.2D   Percent of Operations
Performed Versus Visits >90 Days

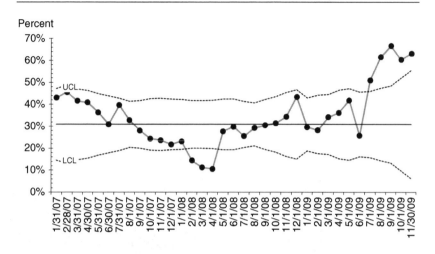

Figure 10.2E   Percent of 19-Year-Olds That Receive Dental Care

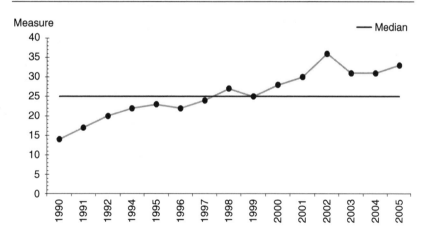

Waiting time has been reduced substantially while improving access to other types of care required by patients. This has been accompanied by an overall drop in the mortality rate in the county. The county council has also won the Swedish Quality Award for four years.

Jönköping County Council provides an excellent example of a leadership team employing the three components discussed in this book:

- Strategic intelligence
- Profound knowledge
- Building a learning organization foundation

In this case study we will discuss each. It should be noted that Jönköping County Council did not have access to the model we call strategic intelligence. However, they have addressed the intent of the model in their application of building a learning organization foundation.

Strategic Intelligence

In chapter 5 we discussed the four components of **strategic intelligence**:

1. Foresight

2. Visioning

3. Motivating

4. Partnering

Foresight

The definition of *foresight* (see Chapter 5) has been described as perception of the significance of events for your organization before they have occurred based on your subject matter expertise, experience, research, scanning, and ability to sense dynamic trends.

The leaders of the organization saw both from demographic data and medical advances that they could expect a higher demand on health care services in the future. They predicted that if they did not control rising costs, they would increase the burden on the tax payers of Jönköping.

Visioning

The leaders of Jönköping developed a systemic vision that can be described in terms of the Four Ps: purpose, practical values, processes, and people.

Figure 10.3 Chain Reaction for Health Care

Improve the system (process, product, service, or system as whole) by which health care is provided

Reduce costs due to less rework, fewer mistakes, delays, patient harm, etc.

Increase patient satisfaction

Improve population health

Note: For the chain reaction to take place a fundamental change must take place as the system is improved. See glossary for fundamental change and the definition of improvement.

Source: Gerald J. Langley, Ronald D. Moen, Kevin M. Nolan, Thomas W. Nolan, Clifford L. Norman, and Lloyd P. Provost, *The Improvement Guide: A Practical Approach to Enhancing Organizational Performance*, 2nd ed. (San Francisco: Jossey-Bass, 2009), Figure 13.2, p. 311.

The purpose of the county council is to provide services of value for the citizens of Jönköping. The system is designed to better serve the health of citizens with continually improving quality and cost.

Sven Olaf, CEO of Jönköping County Council was convinced that focusing on W. Edwards Deming's idea of the **chain reaction** would ensure that quality would be improved while lowering costs. Figure 10.3 describes Deming's Chain Reaction as it relates to a government organization.[3]

To accomplish the chain reaction, the Jönköping County Council Healthcare system would have to be recognized as a system. As the CEO told one of the authors, "We deliver quality care and we must find ways to be more efficient. We need to cause the chain reaction to improve care and reduce costs. I do not want to ask the citizens of my county for more money due to overrunning our budgets."

Health care and nursing should be based on the following practical values:

- Increased availability
- Improved flow of patients and processes in the whole system
- The best possible clinical results with the highest degree of safety
- Implemented at the lowest possible cost

In order to meet these demands Jönköping County Council needed to improve process and develop competent and motivated people.

Motivation

When the work began at Jönköping County Council, the leadership team was not aware of Maccoby's Five Rs of motivation. However, in transforming the organization from viewing itself in silos of hospitals and primary care centers to viewing itself as one system, the Five Rs were addressed. In Chapter 8, the Five Rs were described as

1. Reasons

2. Responsibilities

3. Relationships

4. Recognition

5. Rewards

Reasons

The definition of a leader is someone with followers. The leadership team at Jönköping County Council had followers who believed in the vision. Much of the motivation for focusing on patients came from a case study developed at Jönköping that focused on a Swedish woman named Esther. The Esther story provided a compelling case of an elderly patient in a chronic condition with intermittent acute challenges. The story follows Esther as she arrives at the emergency department after having been seen by the home care nurse. Esther's story highlighted the common errors and delays in the flow and communication as Esther was handed off between professionals and parts of the Jönköping system. Esther put a face on the challenge of providing high-quality and low-cost care to the citizens of Jönköping County Council. Esther became a reason to go to work on improving the system so that patient safety and security would be improved in the future.

Figure 10.4 Understanding the Flow of Patients with Esther

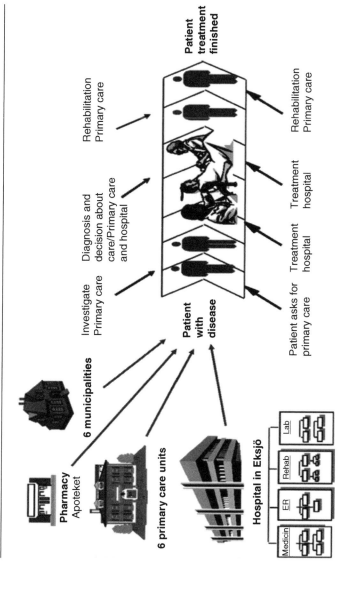

"Esther" is not a real patient: she was invented by the team of physicians, nurses, and other providers who joined together in the Jönköping County Council to improve the way patients flow through the system of care by strengthening coordination and communication among providers. Figure 10.4 describes the role of Esther in understanding the flow of patients.

Everyone at Jönköping County Council was motivated to improve health care for Esther; and to realize the vision the Esther project focused on five overall objectives:

1. Safety for Esther

2. Better working relations

3. Improved competences

4. Improved quality through the entire care chain

5. Improvement documentation and communication

6. Shared medical documentation

These objectives were translated in the action plans in six main projects regarding flexibility of the organization, efficiency of systems, processes, and the use of virtual tools and IT support. This three-year project has resulted in the reduction of hospital admissions and hospital days for patients with heart failure while decreasing waiting times for referral appointments with neurologists and gastroenterologists.

Responsibilities

A primary role of the leader is to place people into meaningful roles that will stimulate intrinsic motivation. We use the word *role* rather than job description to include the opportunity to enhance a person's contribution to the larger system purpose through learning and personal development.

Underlying the idea of the role of the individual and viewing the organization as a system, rather than silos of departments defined by the organization chart, is the notion that *all work is a process*. Given this assumption, each process has workers, process owners, and process experts usually from multiple departments. Not only are responsibilities defined for running the process, but also for understanding how that process impacts the purpose of the system. By focusing on Jönköping County Council as a system, people not only understand their role but how their role interacts and impacts others in the system to contribute to the well-being of the patient. Their intrinsic motivation is engaged as they develop themselves and their roles.

Relationships

The systems view for Jönköping defines the important relationships and interdependences that must be recognized for the system to accomplish its purpose effectively. When faced with challenges to improve, project teams have been encouraged to collaborate. Together they have decided on what would be developed, tested, and implemented based on the overall purpose of the organization.

Recognition

All members of the organization have shared the honor of receiving the Swedish National Award for Quality.

Rewards

As managers transform to leaders, people within the organization are able to see how they relate to and impact the Jönköping Health System. They have learned how to articulate their interdependent roles which are aligned to the Jönköping purpose, holding themselves mutually responsible for achieving improved results. This has created an empowered and rewarding environment in which to grow and learn fueled by intrinsic motivation.

Partnering

The leadership in Jönköping County Council practices partnering in four areas utilizing the center for learning and innovation called **Qulturum**, a local catalyst for regional, national, and also international partnering:

1. Within the leadership team

2. Within the organization

3. Partnering outside Sweden for increasing knowledge

4. Spreading improvement science to other counties in Sweden

The Leadership Team

Sweden celebrates the group. The leadership team at Jönköping included not only the leadership of the health services group, but also the county council leadership. The cooperation between the eighty-one political leaders that make up the council and the leadership of the health care services groups was essential for success. The CEO of Jönköping County Council played a key role in making this partnership work effectively.

When we think of leadership, we sometimes get the visual image of one person leading. The leadership team of the health services group included several people. However three key people were required to partner to cover the leadership role of the system:

- CEO: Sven Olaf
- Qulturum Administrator: Göran Henriks
- Doctor/Administrator of Hospital: Mats Bojestig

Within the leadership team, Sven Olaf, the CEO, provided the authority and the coordination with the county council to take action. Göran Henriks has been especially effective in gathering knowledge from outside the organization to bring back, share, and apply knowledge at Jönköping. Mats Bojestig has partnered with Göran Henriks to bring in new knowledge and to be the communication conduit demonstrating how to apply the new knowledge to physicians and health care professionals within the organization and to the county council.

Within the Organization

The health care services group within Jönköping County Council partners with three groups to ensure leadership and coordination of the entire system.

- The Management Group (MG)
- Big Group Healthcare (BGH)
- Qulturum

THE MANAGEMENT GROUP (MG): A GROUP THAT LEADS AND LEARNS

Focusing on the organization viewed as a system requires coordinated action. The most important task for the MG is to manage care and to administer and develop the system's resources. A strong MG diminishes the risk of suboptimization and fragmentation. Another important task for the MG is to develop and review the system measures and results for the council.

BIG GROUP HEALTHCARE (BGH): THE ARENA OF LEARNING FOR ALL OPERATIONAL HEADS OF DEPARTMENTS

The purpose of the Big Group Healthcare (BGH) is to create an arena of learning for all operational managers and a place where the strategic questions for the county are discussed. These meetings take place five days per year and are led by the head of the county council. A review has shown that one-third of the meeting is about good financing and two-thirds about learning and change. These meetings also help to develop collaboration.

QULTURUM: FOCUSES ON GATHERING AND DISSEMINATING LEARNING FOR THE WHOLE SYSTEM

Qulturum is the county's engine for learning and change with a strategic purpose in the development of individuals to apply learning and achieve improved results for the system. In order to achieve this role, Qulturum is a learning center and meeting point where employees use action-based training in order to improve their respective skills. Qulturum is based on the view that sending people to courses is inadequate; adults learn by doing. Participants have to work with their own challenges from their workplace and "act" into a new way of thinking.

The Qulturum residence also partners with four other entities:

- Apoteket AB (The Swedish Federation of Pharmacies)
- Administration of the county's research and development (R&D)
- Children's health/prevention
- Futurum, the coordination of the clinical practice and research

These partnerships create ties between the delivery of health care and other organizational entities.

Partnering Outside Sweden for Increasing Knowledge

The leadership of the health system in Jönköping County Council has been a great example of leaders who have looked around the world for great ideas to improve patient health in their county.

The leadership of the health care system have been actively involved in sharing and learning at the Institute for Healthcare Improvement[4] since 1997. Each and every year since they have been great contributors at this internationally recognized forum. In addition, they have made visits to health care systems around the world to share and to bring home ideas to test and implement in the county.

Spreading Improvement Science to Other Counties in Sweden

Knowledgeable leadership is needed to carry out the vision and make it successful. To accomplish this aim, leadership needs knowledge in a wide variety of areas. In addition to specific subject matter knowledge relevant to the particular organization, Deming defined the body of knowledge that is necessary for leadership as profound knowledge. As described in Chapter 5, this body of knowledge contains an appreciation of a system, knowledge about variation, psychology, and the theory of knowledge. The system of profound knowledge provides a map of theory to understand and optimize organizations. As Deming explains in the following quotation, a leader does not need to be an expert in all of these areas:

> One need not be eminent in any part of profound knowledge in order to understand it and to apply it. The various segments of the system of profound knowledge cannot be separated. They interact with each other. For example knowledge about psychology is incomplete without knowledge of variation.
>
> The system of profound knowledge provides a lens. It provides a new map of theory by which to understand and optimize our organizations.[5]

A leader should have knowledge of the basic theories in each area, how the different areas interrelate, and why they are important for the improvement and transformation of organizations. Leaders who seek out partners internally and externally with complementary knowledge and skills to leverage and apply these theories create a dynamic rapport for learning and expanding knowledge. Consider three key definitions for our discussion:

Subject matter knowledge: Knowledge basic to the things we do in life; how to ride a bicycle, program a computer, make chemicals, understanding the fundamental physical laws, properties, and scientific theories.

Profound knowledge: The interplay of the theories of systems, variation, knowledge, and psychology.

Science of improvement: Learn to combine subject matter knowledge and profound knowledge in creative ways to develop effective changes for improvement.

Figure 10.5 describes the interplay between these types of knowledge that are necessary to create effective change.

The leadership at Jönköping County Council has been learning about the system of profound knowledge and applying it.

Figure 10.5   Jönköping View of the Interplay Between Professional Knowledge (Subject Matter) and Improvement Knowledge (Profound Knowledge)

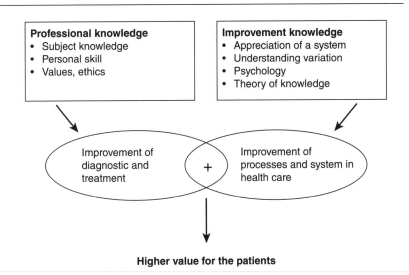

Professional knowledge
- Subject knowledge
- Personal skill
- Values, ethics

Improvement knowledge
- Appreciation of a system
- Understanding variation
- Psychology
- Theory of knowledge

Improvement of diagnostic and treatment
+
Improvement of processes and system in health care

Higher value for the patients

Systems Thinking

Leaders study and manage their organization as a system. They emphasize the importance of common purpose and interdependencies among groups in the organization. They understand that the performance of the organization depends more on the interaction of the various parts than how the parts perform individually. They understand both detail and dynamic complexity in a system. They consider important systems concepts such as boundaries, feedback loops, constraints, and leverage points. They use these concepts to develop, test, and implement changes to accomplish the transformation and better meet the purpose of the organization.

The county council is organized into three health care areas. Each area consists of a hospital with an emergency room and several primary care centers. The challenge for the CEO was to get all three health care areas to view themselves in the same system instead of independent entities. A new picture to supplement the organizational chart was needed to ensure that health care professionals would begin to view themselves in the same system. A conceptual view of this system was drawn by the leadership team to provide a view of Jönköping County Council as "one system." This was a transformation in thinking, moving from a bureaucratic focus on a departmental organization to viewing the organization as one interdependent system focused on patients. Figure 10.6 describes this first conceptual view of the county council viewed as an interdependent system.

The systems view can be divided up into the three areas discussed in Chapter 6: mainstay, driver, and support processes. The mainstay processes describe five major subsystems:

- Access
- Decision support
- Support for self-management
- Delivery of care
- Define ongoing relationships with patients

These five major subsystems are applicable to all primary care centers and all three hospitals. The thirty-five primary care centers

Figure 10.6   Jönköping County Council Viewed as a System

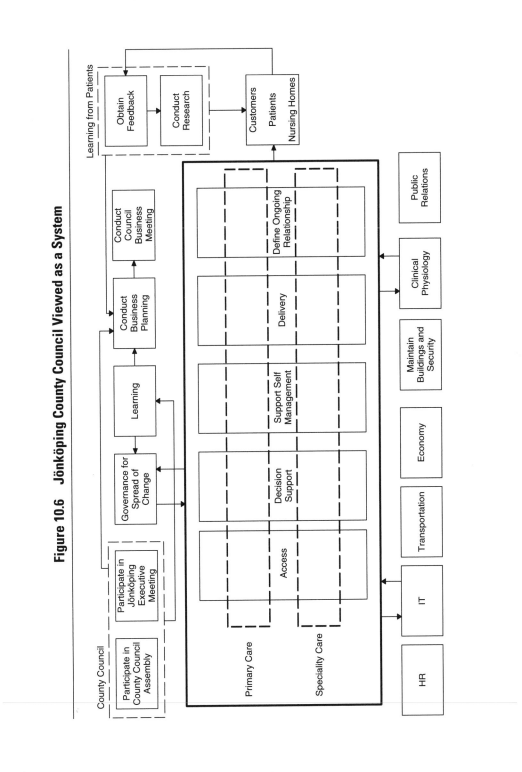

Figure 10.7   CEO Sven Olaf and Big Group Healthcare

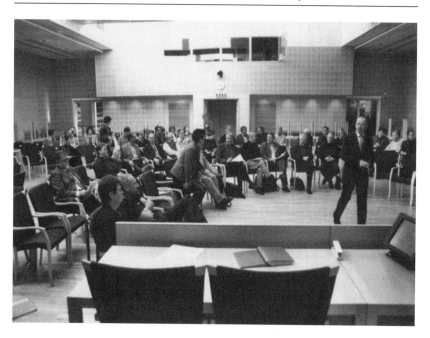

are represented by a horizontal strip that flows across all five major subsystems. The three hospitals are depicted the same way. The CEO was emphatic that the whole system be viewed as one system; patients often had to move between various subsystems. To ensure safety, processes had to be defined that ensured proper handoffs of patients from part of the system to another. As CEO Sven Olaf noted later, "If you are a leader and you are going to lead a system, how do you lead a system without a systems view?" Figure 10.7 shows a picture with the members of the Jönköping leadership team.

Understanding Variation

Leaders understand the different ways that variation is viewed. They explain changes in terms of common causes and special causes. They use graphical methods to learn from data and expect others to consider variation in their decisions and actions. They understand the concept of stable and unstable processes and the

Figure 10.8   Communicating Progress Using Variation Tools

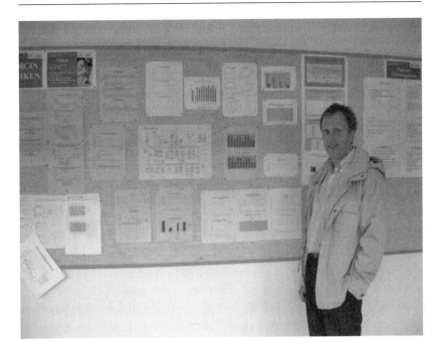

potential losses due to tampering. Thus, the capability of a process or system is understood before changes are attempted.

The leadership team at Jönköping County Council has made an effort to help people understand variation. Workshops have been conducted over several years to develop internal understanding and capability. Graphical tools are used throughout the organization to communicate key measures and the progress of various improvement teams. Figure 10.8 shows Mats Bojestig at a board that describes the progress on various projects. The measures are linked to a systems map of the hospital where Bojestig works.

Theory of Knowledge

Leaders understand that management is prediction that comes from knowledge, and knowledge is built on theory. They understand that people learn in different ways, and they are aware of the importance of judgment heuristics such as representativeness, availability, and anchoring. They use the cycle for learning and improvement to learn, run tests on a small scale, and make decisions. In order to enhance learning, they make predictions before changes are made. They have an understanding of paradigms, mental models, use of paradox, and reframing.

The leaders at Jönköping County Council have learned the importance of the interplay between professional knowledge and profound knowledge. Figure 10.5 describes a view of the relationship between professional knowledge and improvement knowledge.

Psychology

The leaders at Jönköping recognize differences in people and the importance of the fundamental attribution error. They understand the value of teams. They rely more on intrinsic motivation than extrinsic motivation. Resistance to change in their organizations is minimal due to preparation and sharing of information and its meaning in relation to purpose. They plan for the social impact of technical change and make people part of the solution.

The leadership of Jönköping County Council understands that being patient focused requires an emphasis on people; people who receive the care but also the people who deliver the care and support the overall care delivery system. People are encouraged at every level of the health care system to make a contribution to the achievement of the purpose.

Building the Foundation for Learning

The system for learning is built on six methods:

1. Establishing constancy of purpose in the organization

2. Understanding the organization as a system

3. Family of measures (aka, balanced scorecard, dashboard)

4. Designing and managing a system for gathering information for learning

5. Conducting planning for improvement and integrating it with strategic planning

6. Managing and learning from a portfolio of improvement initiatives

These six methods for leaders are focused on aligning an organization on learning so that changes that are developed and implemented move the organization in a desired direction. The methods are interdependent and have to be considered as a system. This approach protects against suboptimization from independently managed individual improvement efforts.

Table 10.2, which outlines methods for **building a system of improvement**, originated from Associates in Process Improvement's

Table 10.2   Methods for Leaders to Build a System of Improvement

Purpose	**Establish and Communicate the Purpose of the Organization**
	• Develop a written statement of purpose of the organization.
	• Include the mission, beliefs, values, and vision.
	• Communicate this purpose to the organization by relating the work of different parts of the organization to the purpose.
	• Use this purpose to guide and focus the business.
Systems Thinking	**View the Organization as a System**
	• Understand the major processes and products in the organization.
	• Document how these processes link together to form a system.
	• Establish the key measures of performance of the system.
	• Use these documents to learn how the organization functions as a system.
Obtaining Information (Customer Focus)	**Establish a System to Obtain Information Relevant to the Need the Information Organization Is Fulfilling**
	• Identify the present and future customers of the organization. Develop a system to gather information concerning needs of customers.
	• Develop systems to obtain other information relevant to the need (from suppliers, employees, marketplace, technology, regulations).
	• Communicate this information to all parts of the organization.
	• Analyze this information to guide planning and improvement efforts.

(continued)

Table 10.2   Continued

Planning	Plan for Improvement
	• Summarize the information from customer research and from employees, suppliers, and the relevant external environment.
	• Based on these inputs, develop (or update) strategic objectives that could best accelerate the performance of the organization.
	• Develop a list in order of priority of the processes, products, and services to design or redesign.
	• Coordinate this plan with the organization's strategic and business planning and budgeting methods.
	• Establish charters to accomplish the improvements that can be resourced and managed.
Managing Improvement	**Manage Individual and Team Improvement Efforts**
	• Provide training and other necessary resources required for the **methods** improvement efforts.
	• Provide a standard methodology to guide improvements.
	• Provide guidance and sponsorship for the team.
	• Remove obstacles and provide recognition.
	• Study the activities of the team to learn about the key processes in the organization and the key forces driving the system.
	• Redirect and redeploy resources as improvements are made.

Quality as a Business Strategy (1993). This has evolved in this case study and those that follow. The evaluation grid in Chapter 11 (Table 11.9) reflects the learning from these case studies, Maccoby's System of Strategic Intelligence, and contributions of other clients, including some outside health care.

The Learning Organization Continues to Learn

Building a system for learning and improvement laid the foundation for Jönköping in creating an organization that learns and adapts. The county council continues its constancy of purpose to

1. Strengthen the ability to focus on results and the things that create value for the customer

2. Develop the support for organizational as well as individual shared learning every day

3. Strengthen the culture with focus on tomorrow

The approaches to learning and innovation are consistent with the Triple Aim:

- Patient's experience of the county's services
- Population's health
- Value for the inhabitants with better productivity and efficiency

For the continuing journey of Jönköping they have developed a picture that describes the Seven Key Questions for organizing for learning from understanding the purpose to integration into every-day work:

1. What is the purpose of our existence?

2. How do we measure our results?

3. How do we define the gap between today and the ideal?

4. How do we develop a connection map to describe the work that is being done?

5. How do we identify waste and links that do not work?

6. How do we prioritize those processes in most need of improvement?

7. How do we integrate improvement work as a natural part of everyday work?

Figure 10.9 describes this journey.

This journey ends with the integration and ownership of improvement into the work of everyone at Jönköping County Council, work that is focused on providing individualized care for each patient. But does the journey end there? Obviously not, as a learning structure has been put in place to ensure that individual learning updates learning for the organization.

Figure 10.9   Seven Questions Showing the Way

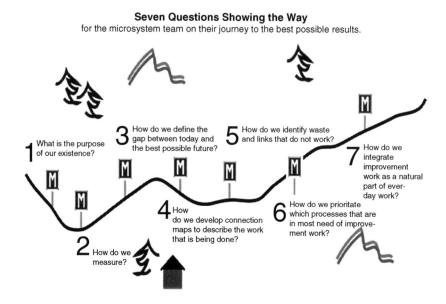

Seven Questions Showing the Way
for the microsystem team on their journey to the best possible results.

1 What is the purpose of our existence?

2 How do we measure?

3 How do we define the gap between today and the best possible future?

4 How do we develop connection maps to describe the work that is being done?

5 How do we identify waste and links that do not work?

6 How do we prioritate which processes that are in most need of improvement work?

7 How do we integrate improvement work as a natural part of everday work?

Summary

Jönköping County Council has provided an excellent example of a leadership team employing the four components necessary for transforming an organization into a learning organization:

- Strategic intelligence
- Leadership philosophy
- Profound knowledge
- Building a foundation for a learning organization

The organization has become an example for health care organizations around the globe to study. By focusing on the patient, Jönköping has provided better access, improved clinical outcomes, lower costs, and dedicated people, results that are sorely needed in health care throughout the world.

CASE STUDY B: A MEDICAL DIRECTOR-LEADER IMPROVES CARE IN DIALYSIS CLINICS

Jerry Jackson is a clinical and interventional nephrologist who serves as the medical director of two dialysis clinics in Birmingham, Alabama.[6] Beginning with his training at the Institute for Healthcare Improvement (IHI) in 2005, he has led an effort to reduce the mortality rate in End Stage Renal Disease patients being treated with hemodialysis. Knowing that there is a strong correlation between the blood level of **albumin** in a hemodialysis patient and the risk of mortality, Jackson decided to take on the challenge of raising the percentage of his hemodialysis patients with a normal albumin level. He has used the components of strategic intelligence, profound knowledge, and the methods of building a system of learning using the science of improvement in his approach to this challenge.

The following narrative describes Jackson's improvement journey in terms of the following outline:

- Strategic intelligence: foresight, visioning, motivating, and partnering
- Profound knowledge: systems thinking, understanding variation, psychology, and theory of knowledge
- Building a foundation for learning: systems map, system measures

Let's begin with foresight, the first component of strategic intelligence.

Foresight

At a workshop for the Network's Medical Review Board leaders, Jackson first heard of the IHI, the Boston-based organization that has become a leader in quality improvement design and training. Having heard how IHI had been instrumental in the design of a program for the end stage renal disease (**ESRD**) program called Fistula First, Jackson wanted to learn more about the science of improvement in hopes of strengthening his efforts to reduce mortality among his patients. He decided to participate in the IHI Improvement Advisers Development Program. In this program, the improvement adviser (IA) has to take a very objective look at all aspects of his or her workplace and then decide on a specific improvement project that will be conducted throughout the IHI workshop. Jackson's project, which began in late 2005, was to attempt to reduce the mortality rate for incident (new) hemodialysis patients. The change package during that phase of his project included

- A new set of tools to guide doctors in the care of patients with advanced chronic kidney disease (CKD) who were expected to need dialysis in the future
- Education of primary care physicians in better care of their own CKD patients
- Use of a nurse practitioner (through a program called RightStart®) to care for new HD patients using a more broad-based approach than typical for these facilities

These activities did result in an improvement in the mortality rate for a group of patients. But there continued to be acute illnesses requiring hospitalization in all the hemodialysis patients, both incident and prevalent patients. In addition, the overall mortality rate continued to be problematic—better than in the past but nonetheless higher than that of Europe and Japan—and so further work was needed.

Shortly after his formal training with IHI, Jackson became more involved with the National Quality Forum, the organization that participates in setting national strategies for health care changes and endorses quality measures for both public reporting and quality improvement. Among many things that Jackson learned from that organization was the concept of *care transitions*. When patients leave one care setting and move to another, the transition is often accompanied with gaps that result in challenges to the patient's health and to specific clinical outcomes. This led Jackson to develop a conceptual framework for the transition that occurs when a hemodialysis patient (both incident and prevalent) leaves a hospital and either starts or resumes care at an outpatient dialysis facility. Very often information from that hospital stay is lacking when the patient returns to the dialysis facility and the dialysis staff has incomplete knowledge of unresolved problems, changes in medications, and new diagnoses. This could possibly lead to further morbidity and mortality, undoing any previous gains in the quality of care.

Jackson had been concentrating on the hospital side of this transition gap in care, developing care modules and hand-off forms that were expected to assist the dialysis staff in delivery of well-informed and better care to the patient once at the facility. Yet he knew that to gain full acceptance of this new care transitions concept among his colleagues, he would have to actually demonstrate a significant improvement in outcomes as a result of a well-designed change in the process of care on the dialysis facility side of the care gap and then link the processes from the hospital side to that of the facility.

In thinking about why some patients die prematurely, Jackson was reminded of what was already known: the major causes were infections and cardiovascular-related death. Whereas objective data about his practice's dialysis population showed generally excellent care in the areas of dialysis delivery, anemia management, vascular access, and control of infections, there were other aspects of care in the hemodialysis clinic population of more concern. These were the problems of accelerated atherosclerosis—both peripheral arterial disease (PAD) and coronary artery disease (CAD)—as well as disorders of bone-mineral metabolism (such as hyperparathyroidism, hyperphosphatemia and hypercalcemia that very likely resulted in arterial calcification). In addition, protein-energy malnutrition (PEM) seemed to be an ongoing severe problem that greatly affected the average patient's quality of life. Low albumin level (hypoalbuminemia) has long served as a marker for this PEM and in fact was a severe problem in his clinics.

Based on his work as chairman of the Medical Review Board of NW8, Jackson knew that this was in fact a widespread problem and one that had resisted change for well over a decade despite significant nutritional interventions.

Jackson decided that albumin outcomes would be a most challenging clinic outcome measure to improve. If an improvement could be made through the well-established quality improvement techniques he had been taught, it might cause other nephrologists to use these methods. When Jackson reviewed the existing literature on causes of hypoalbuminemia, he discovered that what was already well reported in the literature was not being utilized widely in the practice of dialysis care. He learned that there is a strong correlation between low albumin level and higher mortality risk in this population of patients. This mortality seems to be from cardiovascular disease, likely with the same biological pathways that caused the low albumin level also causing the accelerated atherosclerosis. Inflammation and oxidative stress seemed too often to be a common pathway for both PEM and accelerated atherosclerosis.

The in-depth literature review was instrumental in leading Jackson to design a set of interventions, with multiple factors at low and high levels used according to the needs of the individual patient on a month-by-month basis. As broadly defined in the Hasting Center's report, his interventions were considered a quality improvement project and not clinical research in the traditional sense. The following characteristics of the project as conceptualized and then conducted fit with the criteria as set forth in that document for a quality improvement project:

- All patients were under Jackson's direct management
- All interventions had evidence-based support in peer-reviewed medical journals
- There were no control groups
- Therapies were individualized and changed over time according to each patient's ongoing needs

However, Jackson needed to explain his learning to the others in the organization to gain and enlist their full support. The potential importance of improving the dialysis facility's average albumin level was explained to key workers in a regularly scheduled quality review committee. The Centers for Medicare & Medicaid Service (CMS) has oversight of these dialysis facilities, and recently a revised Conditions for Coverage document was produced by CMS to guide facilities in proper management and to clarify regulatory oversight. As part of this, it was mandated that each facility conduct quality assurance and process improvement projects, supervised by the medical director of that facility. Jackson presented the case that improvement of albumin would be a perfect example of this type of project, since this was a metric that had not improved over a very long time despite a top-down management approach largely oriented around a nutritional approach. Improvement of albumin could potentially have a beneficial impact on reduction of morbidity and mortality among the patient population for whom both the medical director and the facility's corporate owner through its staff were charged to provide care. Other key members of this team would be the facility dietician, its social worker, and its nurse manager. All were very enthusiastic and have since proven themselves to be partners in the project. The goal would be to show a significant improvement in the percent of patients cared for in the facility with a monthly Alb level of 4.0 gm% or above. This in fact has been a metric used in dialysis care since the late 1990s under the Core Indicators project by CMS.

Motivating

Jackson's alignment with the Five Rs of motivation was very apparent in this case:

- *Reasons:* Obvious patient care and compliance with required efforts from CMS.
- *Relationships:* The dietician and the social worker round with Jackson (the medical director and clinical nephrologist) on each patient each month in order to know the exact state of the change package as applied to that patient and to participate in the areas of their own specialty training. The nurse manager operated primarily in a facilitating role.
- *Responsibilities:* When the social worker and dietician round with the Jackson on each patient on a monthly basis, they discuss the status of the parameters as determined to potentially play a role in that person's Alb level and decide on the portions of the overall change package that should be applied to that individual for the next month. They follow up on those interventions to ensure compliance and effectiveness. The nurse manager facilitates information flow and gives feedback on corporate clinic level data as it is reported.
- *Rewards:* Enthusiasm and intrinsic motivation of each member of the team for the project is remarkable and this has been sustained over time. Each person is a true professional in their specialty and receives gratification in seeing the effectiveness of the interventions in terms of the improvement in the facility's numeric rating for Alb levels but also in the improved wellness of the individual patients under their charge. The improvement in an area where such improvement had not previously occurred also gains them respect from colleagues.
- *Recognition:* Clinics are compared nationally and as this clinic is recognized as a leader, all will share in the recognition.

Partnering

At the dialysis facility level, the key partnership is with the three staff members as well as with each individual patient.

- The dietician has a critical role in deriving the numeric equivalent of the patient's protein intake, a number needed in the determination of the specific intervention needed for that month. The group of patients as a whole have a below average socioeconomic position and need the assistance of the social worker in order to fully participate in a number of aspects of the recommended treatments inherent in the change package.
- The nurse manager is essential in tracking the overall facility scores and reporting back to corporate, as well as in keeping a record of the progress for external surveys needed for accountability.
- The medical director is the leader of the project as well as the individual primary nephrologist for each involved patient. As such, Jackson determines which order set to write for each patient on a monthly basis. In addition, and most important, he maintains a doctor-patient relationship with each individual being cared for in the clinics involved in this project and uses this role for encouragement and education of the patient to gain their cooperation.

Use of Profound Knowledge

Systems Thinking

Conceptually, it occurred to Jackson that each patient is a unique individual, with a cause system for low albumin level that is different from the other patients. Over time, even a single patient can have changing primary causes for low albumin. So the scrutiny of that individual patient over time is critical to the correct application of the change package. Only as individual patients show improvement will the facility average albumin level improve. So while the facility's percentage of patients with normal albumin is the metric by which the clinic is judged, an across the board, top-down management protocol that treats all patients the same will be (and in fact has been) doomed to failure. With that in mind, a conceptual approach emerged based on the idea of stacked systems where each system consists of its set of interacting processes, then with layers of systems above the lower system. And vertical interactions exist between each layered system. The system above the base (patient) system is the facility, with its mainstay processes as well as driver and support processes. Then the level is the corporate ownership system that drives down corporate policies, procedures and protocols. Finally, above that system is the containing system, the ESRD Program of CMS with its set of regulations and guidance.

The important part of this concept is that the single patient, an individual human being, is in fact a system (Figure 10.10) that consists of biological, psychological, environmental, and spiritual processes. These processes all interact in a way to affect outcomes, such as baseline levels of things such as albumin and also responsiveness to various treatments, to dietary intake, and even the will to live. It is inconceivable that a single protocol driven from above could apply to all people in a care system and that a stable outcome or response could result. Thus the concept of individual patient as a system was foundational for this project.

Figure 10.10   Patient as a System Nested in the Care Delivery System

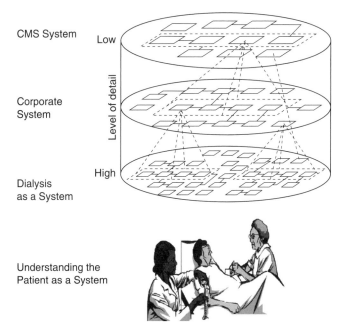

Source: Gerald J. Langley, Ronald D. Moen, Kevin M. Nolan, Thomas W. Nolan, Clifford L. Norman, and Lloyd P. Provost, *The Improvement Guide: A Practical Approach to Enhancing Organizational Performance*, 2nd ed. (San Francisco: Jossey-Bass, 2009).

Understanding Variation

A robust database of monthly albumin level for each patient was established. Additionally, individual patient characteristics as well as intervention factors with their levels were charted. Then the percent of the entire population with an albumin reaching target level (4.0 gm% or above) was charted by month and a run chart applied. Retrospective baseline data for six months prior to the implementation of the change package was added to the database and the subsequent eighteen months of data during the time of interventions was entered. The total patient population during this time consisted of eighty-five individuals. During this time, new patients entered the facilities while patients left due to kidney recovery, transplantation, transfer to home dialysis or another inpatient facility, or death. This created the situation of a moving stream of data, with the population ever-changing over time. This "stock and flow" situation lent itself much better to analytic type statistical treatments than the more traditional enumerative statistics characteristic of biomedical research with its randomized controlled trials.

Figure 10.11 demonstrates a significant (at the 95 percent confidence interval) improvement with this change package as compared to the baseline data.

Figure 10.11   Run Chart with Albumin Target of 4.0 or Above

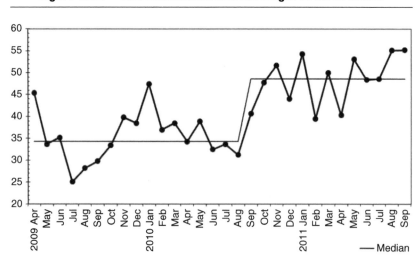

Knowledge

Jackson employed the Model for Improvement in this project. The three questions of the model have given guidance to ensure a focus on the principle aim and that changes would result in achieving the defined measures. Question three lays out the journey of the project: what changes can we make that will result in improvement? The **project charter** in Exhibit 10.1 describes the use of the Model for Improvement for the Albumin Project.

Psychology

Each patient was visited each month for two years and careful assessment was carried out each visit, with revision of the change package potentially each month. Then the data was faithfully recorded and validated so that the analytic study would be meaningful. In addition, there was an excellent doctor-patient relationship that resulted in the patient believing that the doctor was conducting these interventions for his or her best interests. A caring approach, with careful explanation of the rationale for each phase of the intervention was critical. It is difficult to say whether the improvement could be spread to different environments with different doctors and patients without this level of attention to detail and caring for the patient. In addition, it was essential that the doctor-leader have a positive relationship with the other team members. They had to sustain a belief that the system of care was worth the effort applied, with confidence that went beyond the immediate response as a considerable time lag existed between intervention and results. Confidence, belief, hope, and patience were personality characteristics important for all participants.

■ EXHIBIT 10.1: MODEL FOR IMPROVEMENT: ALBUMIN PROJECT CHARTER

1. What are we trying to accomplish? To increase the percentage of patients in the dialysis facility with serum albumin $=>4.0$ by at least 50 percent.

2. How will we know that a change is an improvement?

    - Outcome Measure:
      Percentage of patients with Alb $=$ or > 4.0 over time

- Process Measures:
  Percent referral for specific inflammatory cause

  Percent use of anti-inflammatory medications

  Percent achieving ideal dialysis prescription

  Percent achieving ideal protein dietary intake
- Balancing Measures:
  Cost per patient

  Patient satisfaction

3. What changes can we make that will result in improvement?

- Correct and control metabolic acidosis
- Ensure that the intra-dialytic weight gain (fluid accumulation) is less than 3.0 kg
- Ensure that the patient with low albumin has fully adequate dialysis over the duration of dialysis = to or > 4 hr
- Ensure that the patient's protein intake is adequate as indicated by nPNA = 1.0–1.2
- Identify and then intervene to correct any and all detectable underlying specific conditions responsible for high inflammatory state
- Categorize the patient according to level of inflammatory state according to the level of C-reactive protein and use appropriate interventions for that category
- Removal of central venous catheters, remnant AVGs, or rejected renal transplants as possible and as indicated
- Use of Sevelamer as indicated for hyperphosphatemia
- Use of ACE inhibitors for hypertension if the patient has elevation in C-reactive protein
- Use of a statin drug if the patient has elevation in LDL
- Use of vitamin C and vitamin E for nonspecific inflammatory state

---

Building a System for Learning

Jackson and the team aligned and focused on the patient using the following two key components of a system for learning:

1. Purpose of the organization

2. Systems view of the dialysis clinic

Each component will be described and supported with specific examples from Jackson's clinics.

1. Purpose of the Dialysis Clinic:

Patients with ESRD carry an unusually high burden of illness that leads to physical and psychological instability, extra personal and family stresses, and extra financial obligations. As providers of care to the individual with ESRD we will strive to provide care that is safe, efficient, timely, equitable, effective, and patient-centered (see Figure 10.12).

Figure 10.12   Hypoalbuminemia: Related Conditions and Care Across Time for ESRD Patients on HD

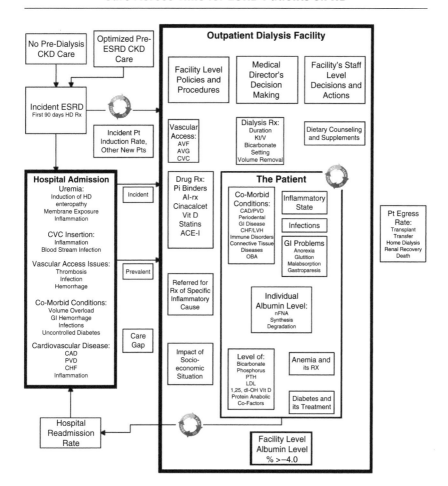

The Albumin Project is aimed directly at the core of this purpose statement; improvement from this project will contribute greatly to being patient centered while improving the safety and efficiency of care that is effective clinically.

2. System Maps:

Jackson was instrumental in defining the clinic as a system. Nested within the dialysis clinic viewed as a system is how the patient interacts between the hospital and the dialysis clinic. The symbol of the PDSA cycle describes the number of improvement changes underway during the Albumin Project. Figure 10.12 describes this system flow.

Summary

This project was originally conceived as a project nested within a larger set of projects designed with the goal of reduction in mortality of incident (or new, first 90 days) hemodialysis patients who were being cared for in outpatient dialysis facilities. It was an outgrowth of the concept of care transitions. Any of a number of subsets of a larger project on improving the care transitions of a patient going from a hospital to a dialysis facility could have been chosen as the next in line for improvement. Hypoalbuminemia being such a historically difficult parameter to change within a hemodialysis population made this parameter both a challenge and an opportunity useful to demonstrate the techniques described in this section. However, over the course of the project, this view has been modified and expanded.

Typical of successful quality improvement projects, things are learned that were not previously obvious to the team conducting the quality improvement (QI) effort, and indeed many things were learned. That albumin could be improved to the degree such that these clinics have been recognized as being in the 97–100 percentile of all clinics in the nation for this parameter taught that remarkable progress can be made with well-conducted QI techniques, assuming that those involved are given the proper time and resources to carry the project through to its true completion. In this regard, short-term return on investment can be considered the enemy of such projects. So often, time lags occur for multiple reasons between the implementation of a change package and the ultimate benefit. Another level of learning was the awareness of how a parameter such as albumin can relate to so many different subsystems within both the human biologic system and the dialysis care system. Improvement in hypoalbuminemia has truly been recognized as a "high leverage point." Jackson's team learned that being below normal always had some cause or multiple causes, and that the cause or causes being detected would be of ultimate benefit to the patient. And early in the project the team realized that the project applied to all of the facilities' patients, not just the new (incident) patients. It was beyond the scope of this project to clearly define whether or not this improvement in prevailing albumin levels would indeed result in reduced mortality rates, but that is clearly the hope and even expectation. And further iterations of the improvements as well as additions to the change package are being considered.

An additional insight was that much more could be learned by subgrouping the data and using graphical displays (run charts and control charts), rather than looking at all data pooled together in tables. By dividing the patients into subgroups of low, medium, and high levels of inflammation, more rational bundles of change implementations can be designed and applied to each subgroup.

It is worth noting that a project such as this meets the well intended regulations by CMS that promote such work and are aimed at improved patient outcomes and well-being. Also, by participating as a team at the facility level, the involved physician and the facility's staff are bonded in a joint sense of purpose that enhances their own professional goals and satisfaction. Finally, this project resulted in a very strong growth in the doctor-patient relationship in these facilities, with the sense among the patients that their well-being has been paramount in the design and conduct of the improvement effort.

This project is an example of a physician-led improvement project with a small and highly centralized team, with tight focus applied over a fairly lengthy timeframe. It was notable in that the more traditional concepts of the doctor-patient relationship and evidence-based medicine were blended with formal quality improvement techniques to form an implementation design that resulted in extremely good results.

CASE STUDY C: BUILDING A LEARNING ORGANIZATION AT OCHIN, PORTLAND, OREGON, UNITED STATES

Background

The original CEO of a payer organization demonstrated foresight when she proposed and submitted a grant to the United States Federal government in 1999 to coordinate and provide electronic medical records to their member clinics in order to reduce costs in processing claims while creating a database which would be used to improve patient care and community health. In 2000, she received a small grant to plan and begin implementation of this idea.

The leadership team formed the Oregon Community Healthcare Information Network (OCHIN) with their community clinic partners to evaluate, choose, configure, and install electronic medical record software. The partner collaborative selected EPIC as the software solution that would best fit their needs for the present and the future. It is interesting to note that EPIC was the first software to be certified in 2010 by the U.S. federal government agency (Office of the National Chairman [ONC]), charged to define and provide incentives for health care entities to install electronic medical records under the Obama Affordable Care Act. In 2005, the current executive group divested their information technology network and OCHIN became an independent organization.

Strategic Intelligence

As OCHIN embarked as an independent entity, the leadership group defined their purpose as "providing technology information and solutions to the medically underserved." Their core work was to configure and install EPIC systems to nonprofit community clinics. OCHIN eventually was given the license to configure and host EPIC software for the unique billing and local reporting requirements for community clinics throughout the United States allowing them to expand their network of members outside of Oregon. Soon OCHIN expanded to Oregon, Washington, and California and was receiving inquiries from communities in Midwestern and Eastern states. As their membership base expanded beyond Oregon, they redefined OCHIN as "Our" Community Healthcare Information Network.

The original funding for OCHIN came from Health Resources and Services Administration (HRSA) federal grants to research, install and host EPIC. As OCHIN grew, they continued in a traditional manner to expand the business in software support. For example, many clinics have limited resources to hire billing expertise to resolve claim and billing issues. As a result, OCHIN began contracting with members to manage claims and accounts receivable.

OCHIN routinely partners with state and community entities. These parties encouraged OCHIN to apply to the federal government for a Regional Extension Center for Oregon. For CEO Abby Sears (OCHIN's first employee), this direction would move OCHIN closer to the foresight of the original CEO who formed OCHIN not just to install and support electronic medical records but to reduce costs in processing claims while creating a database which would be used to improve patient care and community health.

OCHIN was ready to move beyond being an EPIC hosting, configuration, installation, and support organization. As the EPIC host, they had the database, and members who joined OCHIN shared EPIC software solutions. The OCHIN membership permeated Oregon with an existing learning network and trust relationship that could be used to improve patient care and community health. Soon all members in seven states were able to see medical records of any patient in the system if they moved or were in an emergency situation. OCHIN was already working with members to utilize the database for better care of patients with a product called Solutions that data-mined health care data in a usable format for health care professionals to empanel and provide better patient care. The objective of the Federal Regional Extension Centers was in total alignment to the existing networking structure at OCHIN. It seemed logical for OCHIN to submit a Regional Extension Center grant proposal, which would serve not only OCHIN's existing nonprofit community clinics but also for-profit clinics, small hospitals with less than ten beds, and small private practices with less than ten doctors.

Purpose

In preparation for the future, OCHIN began a major effort to examine its purpose and vision by reexamining its products, services, delivery system, and personnel by focusing on creating a learning environment. During the journey that will be described below, the need to revise their organizational purpose became evident as they expanded both their member base and their products and services. In 2011, the board approved a revised mission to expand and align to the newly designed system and members.

OCHIN Mission (*purpose* in our context)

2009—Providing technology information and solutions to the medically underserved

2011—Partnering with communities to create the knowledge and information solutions to promote access to high-quality and affordable health care for all

The Journey

In December of 2009, the executive leadership team, senior leadership team, and employee representatives used the **Quality as a Business Strategy (QBS)** evaluation grid (basis for the evaluation grid—strategic intelligence and Four Ps in Chapter 11) to identify gaps and opportunities during a strategic retreat. As a result, OCHIN began a transformation to a learning organization, by focusing on the gap analysis and methods provided by the original Quality as a Business Strategy evaluation grid. Their journey started in earnest in 2010 by focusing on the alignment of their purpose and vision to the system.

Aligning Purpose and Vision to the System

Because they were redesigning the mainstay or delivery system, OCHIN initially utilized their existing mission (*purpose* in our context) to begin redesigning their system using the system map. However, work had been done to create a system map of how work was currently done. Here is the original conceptual framework of the OCHIN delivery system with two primary subsystems (see Figure 10.13):

The natural inclination was to simplify and standardize the subsystem that included most of OCHIN's resources: configuration and installation of EPIC software. But Sears recognized the system map was incomplete. Refining the installation processes would not fulfill the needs of the existing members. Sears needed a way to help people see the new OCHIN and membership in a different light.

Figure 10.13   Original Conceptual Framework of the OCHIN Delivery System with Two Subsystems

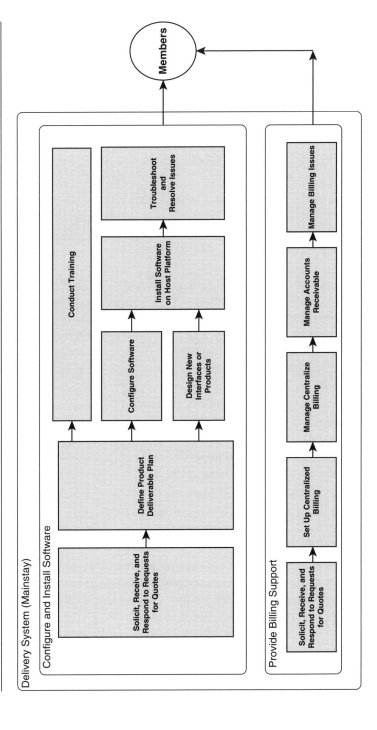

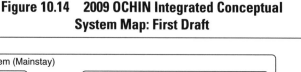

Figure 10.14   2009 OCHIN Integrated Conceptual System Map: First Draft

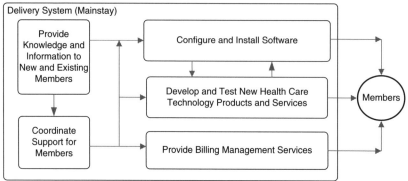

Vision

Sears described her vision for OCHIN explicitly as a collaborative learning organization which encompasses the whole system, assisting health care providers with data analysis and tools for effective and efficient patient and community care once any electronic health care record system was installed. She acknowledged that resources were being sucked up by the installation process and focus on new members. The constraints of the past were to be put aside to design new and redesign old processes that would leverage strengths and knowledge within the ranks. Figure 10.14 shows the mainstay framework that was initially created from the dialogue that ensued, expanding from two subsystems to five to allow additional products and services.

Redesigning the System

In January 2010, OCHIN was named the Regional Extension Center for Oregon by the newly defined ONC which was charged to define and act as the officiating group for the new Affordable Care Act's Center for Medicare & Medicaid Services (CMS). The objective was to install electronic medical records throughout the nation by giving physicians financial incentives to not only install but also use the data for improvement of care to patients. They coined the term *meaningful use* of health care data with a complex tier. Funding would be dependent on the number of qualifying members with signed agreements with each Regional Extension Center. Although Regional Extension Center grants were awarded in January, the document for defining and qualifying members, incentives, and structural guidelines was not defined by the government until late summer. At least 25 percent of members originally defined when the grants were written were disqualified by late summer of 2010.

OCHIN was renamed the Oregon Regional Extension Center O-HITEC. There was no government model to follow, only expected results to deliver. OCHIN was ready for the transformation since the new conceptual delivery system defined how work would flow and the interdependencies. All of these subsystems would be necessary for O-HITEC. While other Regional Extension Centers were focused primarily on the installation of electronic medical record programs and trying to sell them, O-HITEC was looking at developing an integrated system. Five subsystems were integrated into the delivery system, with three new subsystems to focus their execution:

1. Providing knowledge and information to new and existing membership (which expanded beyond EPIC requests for quotes)

2. Coordinating member support

3. Developing and testing new health care products and services

Manpower was immediately added to the first subsystem to develop and execute processes to provide knowledge and information to new and existing members. This group designed educational sessions, a new website, and solicited information from potential new members into the O-HITEC incentive system to help identify their needs. An installed certified EMS was the base requirement of the incentive system. EPIC was predicted to be one of the certified systems. Therefore, physicians in the OCHIN membership would automatically qualify for the first year's incentive, but that was not sufficient to meet the first year's quota for O-HITEC. Small private practices and small hospitals that had a defined percentage of Medicare/Medicaid patient populations were the qualifying group. The cost of EPIC was prohibitive for most small practices and OCHIN was not authorized to install EPIC in small hospitals. O-HITEC would leverage OCHIN's strength, configuring and installing electronic health record (**EHR**). But they needed to assess other products and get feedback from potential members. Currently installation capabilities have expanded to include Allscripts EHR, eClinicalWorks EHR, addition authorization for EPIC applications in hospitals with fewer than ten beds, and recently Greenway's PrimeSuite EHR. All products include secure health information exchange capabilities and web-based patient portals that let patients and doctors communicate easily, safely, and securely over the Internet.

All products offered by OCHIN are geared to enable members and clients to implement and achieve meaningful use of their EHR as required to secure federal incentive payments and support provider and practice efforts to advance clinical, financial, and operational goals—the preconditions for clinical transformation.

The intent of installing electronic health records goes beyond input of a patient's data by the health care provider. Expanding from an internal system's view to responding to the needs of clinics, health care professionals, and all users and potential patients has enabled OCHIN to expand services to include

1. *Business Services* provides multitiered support designed to create operational efficiencies and drive savings directly into OCHIN-supported practices.

2. *Data Services* provides the capability to aggregate data from any number of vendor sources enabling users to interface with, and build on, existing clinical, financial, and operational tools already in place for reporting and improving health outcomes. OCHIN's data warehouse is tailored to a health care environment and uses an innovative proprietary data aggregation architecture that makes the accurate measurement of clinical and operational variables straightforward, thus making it possible to compare metrics easily across different organizations without the need for complicated audits. All data exchange is governed by agreements that are compliant with applicable laws and regulations governing protected health information.

3. *Health Information Exchange* (HIE) connects all OCHIN network members via Epic Care Everywhere network that connects hospitals nationally and through the emerging Nationwide Health Information Network (NwHIN) exchange. OCHIN is also building a national HIE capability that utilizes the rules and guidelines for how computer systems should exchange information defined by Health Level Seven International (HL7) with the international Integrating the Healthcare Enterprise (IHE) initiative for health care–specific data. These solutions enable OCHIN to seamlessly integrate multiple systems including hospital registration systems, laboratory systems, immunization registries, and, via the NwHIN, to support information exchange with federal agencies. Using OCHIN, administrative and clinical staff can coordinate patient care across multiple states and unrelated health care entities, giving care providers the knowledge to improve patient outcomes regardless of where patient treatment took place.

4. *Practice-Based Research Network* (PBRN) operates as an independent business unit within OCHIN for the purpose of encouraging practice-based research that advances understanding of the health of underserved populations, increases health equity, improves quality of care, and informs health policy. The OCHIN PBRN is unique among other practice-based research networks because it has no formal affiliation with a particular academic health center and is comprised almost exclusively of federally qualified health centers (FQHCs) and rural health centers (RHCs).

The evolution of the OCHIN system map has expanded to show these important subsystems and their integration to achieve the organization's purpose. Systems thinking continues to drive the organization to solicit and assess member and patient needs. PDSA symbols have been added to the OCHIN system map to reflect where internal prioritized Accelerated Model for Improvement projects (Ami™ charters) are targeted. In addition, OCHIN is using their system map as part of their analysis, prioritization, resource allocation, and communication of joint improvement projects initiated by members' requests to address growing member and patient documentation and analysis needs (see Figure 10.15).

Figure 10.15 2012 OCHIN Conceptual System Map with Internal and Member Ami™ Improvement Projects

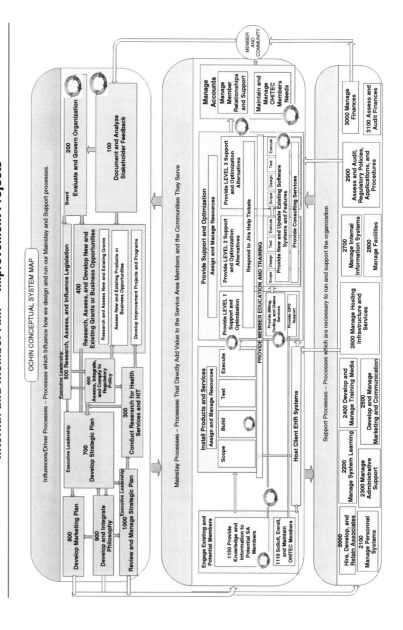

Using Personality Intelligence in a Changing Environment

Early in 2009, OCHIN began using the Strength Deployment Inventory (SDI) from Personal Strengths Publishing as a means to educate and develop personality intelligence throughout OCHIN. Assessment of the 2009 delivery processes using the new system maps revealed some interesting issues. First, the billing subsystem had only one manager, Phil Skiba. He was an experienced manager who had executive experience at larger companies with a strong personality to get things done and a willingness to make changes, while routinely treating risk as a challenge. Skiba was also aware that his strong personality had to be held back when working with more analytic and nurturing personalities, which was the predominant cultural norm. He used his SDI learning to modify his communication methods to improve relationships and communications. In a relatively short time, he had taken the small subsystem over and grown it with more clients, delivering excellent results for these billing customers.

In contrast, the install subsystem was composed of six managers. Five of them had been promoted from within, with no management experience nor any management or leadership training. They were in a high-stress environment and were constantly adapting and making changes to make things work. But some changes were not aligned with strategic plans, which forced them to make additional changes. This only created more stress and confusion. Their flexible-adaptive personality profiles explained this behavior. In a rapidly growing and changing organization, management needs alignment and experienced leadership.

By the end of 2009, the decision was made to begin the transition to test the revised delivery system. Within weeks, OCHIN was officially informed that they had been selected as the Oregon Regional Extension Center, renamed O-HITEC. Realigning resources to move toward the new integrated delivery system was critical for success. Five managers were moved back into the organization for added delivery resources. Experienced leaders within the organization were reassigned. The previous COO, Clayton Gillett, now became the designated leader of the O-HITEC group and was assigned to develop and integrate the processes to provide knowledge and information to new and existing members. The existing quality assurance director was moved to coordinating support for members. Skiba (a certified project manager) retained billing but was allowed to hire a billing manager so that he could also manage the project managers for the installation processes. The new COO, Jane Norman, managed personnel for EPIC configuration and development of new products and services.

OCHIN began a series of communication sessions with their associates, many of whom had been with the organization from the beginning. Initially, the leadership team delegated communication to the COO, who conducted weekly meetings. Later the executive leadership team took ownership. Leadership predicted weekly meetings and openness in these meetings would help the associates make the transition.

With the announcement of O-HITEC, the new delivery system was unveiled. The first stage reallocated leadership responsibilities. These were shared using the revised delivery system map with leaders' names noted in the next stage. Demand in the subsystems was assessed to begin a transition of people for dedicated resources. Roles had not been determined, but would be shortly. In order to do this without disrupting the installation process, OCHIN's primary financial resource, some programmers would work in two subsystems for the first few months. In an effort to dispel anxiety that changes were permanent, leadership stated that the delivery system was like Jell-O—as we mold it, we will review it. Changes that were not working would be abandoned and a new mold would be created from what was learned.

The leadership team was committed to learning from experience and making necessary changes. Skepticism that the delivery system would never be more than an installation effort flowed from side conversations spreading skepticism to others who had been optimistic. Communication and transparency was essential. As Mark Twain once noted, "A lie can travel halfway around the world while the truth is still putting on its shoes." In addition, the COO learned at the second communication session that the Jell-O analogy was causing anxiety. She was a flexible-adaptive personality who was comfortable with uncertainty and learning from changes. But for the analytic and nurturing programmers, Jell-O communicated uncertainty. They needed specific direction. They wanted to be told what to do and that the plan was solid.

The Jell-O analogy was abandoned. The COO replaced it with another analogy of "building the bridge as we walk on it" and stated that the framework of most of the bridge was already in place. O-HITEC would take the response to quotes, define additional processes, and integrate into subsystem 1. Subsystem 2 was putting new processes in place for the informal help desk. Subsystem 3 was dedicating more resources to new products like Solutions, which was already in place. More resources for O-HITEC and the delivery system would be added. Developing processes and roles were the next hurdles. Throughout the transition everyone was responsible for learning and sharing knowledge. The new analogy and explanation of the new delivery system, "building the bridge," soon became a common theme. And leadership learned more about personality intelligence and the communication needs of the organization.

Using Role Descriptions to Integrate People into the Learning Organization

Starting in 2007, OCHIN doubled its members and the number of visits hosted yearly. When OCHIN had under twenty people, it was easy to learn from one another. But in 2009, with sixty-two people, it became harder to facilitate learning. Once the revised delivery system was in place, the organization was flattened with existing and new resources allocated to the five major interdependent subsystems of the delivery system. The initial restructuring of existing resources in the five subsystems exposed other weaknesses in the system, specifically personnel with underdeveloped skills and those who were doing more than their share of work to make up for the inadequacies of others. What skills did individuals need to be successful? How could OCHIN leverage and utilize individuals' strengths and knowledge?

In 2009, approximately one-third of the staff were application specialists whose skills were critical for the success of support, installation, and new products, or 60 percent of the delivery subsystems. These skills were developed in three main categories: basic structure, clinical, and billing. There was no master skill list for training or assessing application specialist's knowledge or skills. Leadership worked with subject matter experts to define 100 skills for each of the three skill categories. Skills were self-assessed by each of the application specialists using a similar format to the portion of the form below. This helped define what an application specialist knew. The list has since been refined to 122 skills in seventeen areas. In addition, 53 skills for training members in EPIC functions have been defined in five areas to assess and develop application trainers' skill levels. Figure 10.16 describes the Skills Assessment Tools Format.

Figure 10.16 Skills Assessment Tools Format

Application Specialist - Skills Assessment   Name:

5 Skills — Coaching, Facilitation, and Presentation

| | Demonstrated Skill Level | | | | |
Skills ID / Skill Description	Expert (Ability to Troubleshoot)	Intermediate (Seldom needs help)	Basic (With Written Process)	Education Only	No Experience

17 Skills — Prelude Build and Configure Structure

| | Demonstrated Skill Level | | | | |
Skills ID / Skill Description	Expert (Ability to Troubleshoot)	Intermediate (Seldom needs help)	Basic (With Written Process)	Education Only	No Experience

8 Skills — Configure Provider Master File Build

| | Demonstrated Skill Level | | | | |
Skills ID / Skill Description	Expert (Ability to Troubleshoot)	Intermediate (Seldom needs help)	Basic (With Written Process)	Education Only	No Experience

13 Skills — Configure Security Build

| | Demonstrated Skill Level | | | | |
Skills ID / Skill Description	Expert (Ability to Troubleshoot)	Intermediate (Seldom needs help)	Basic (With Written Process)	Education Only	No Experience

34 Skills — EpicCare Build

| | Demonstrated Skill Level | | | | |

Based on the results, each application specialist was classified by skills in one of four categories: basic structure, clinical, billing, or training. For each category a technical lead (who had demonstrated the highest knowledge) was identified. The leads were charged with conducting learning sessions and utilizing the skills inventory to build the skills of their technical group. Fridays were declared learning days to support the time needed to develop the skills. As application specialists mastered and demonstrated new skills, salaries were adjusted.

The skills inventories also became a tool for hiring experienced individuals. Candidates self-assessed their skills, and if they passed the previous screening interviews, a technical lead interviewed them to verify their skill levels.

Additional technical leads were identified throughout the organization and Friday learning days were used for sharing learning during the week. Helping the technical leads learn the difference between telling or managing people and leading and developing people was a challenge. A three-day leadership workshop at Gettysburg was conducted by Austin API, Inc., with follow-up sessions for learning. Primarily the executive leadership team attended. Attendees used the experience to learn, reflect with one another, and become better leaders. A key lesson from experience is *courage*, which was discussed in Chapter 8. On the battlefield a leader must display physical courage. In business, the effective leader must display moral courage and be prepared to move beyond the second level of ethics and morality discussed in Chapter 4 to a third level, where the leader and team might have to sacrifice for the overall system. The following year, a second group of technical leads and additional managers attended the three-day Gettysburg leadership experience. These learning sessions were building leaders at all levels within OCHIN and creating a learning environment with a shared understanding of the three levels of ethics and morality necessary to support the practical values of OCHIN.

The skills inventory (including training) for different levels of application specialists requires understanding the processes a role performs and the knowledge needed to be effective. Traditional job descriptions focus on reporting structure, pay scales, qualifications and generalized skills. Formal role descriptions are a critical tool to align individuals and develop them within a learning organization.

Role descriptions have been developed for all associates and have replaced job descriptions. They are currently used for yearly individual development plans. Processes and the skills required were used to define the role descriptions, so that organizational pay grades were matched with market levels, but also demonstrated expertise. In addition to traditional job description information the role description explicitly states the following additions (see Role Description Template in Exhibit 10.2):

1. How the role contributes to the purpose of the organization

2. The processes in which the individual is expected to execute

3. Measures of the process to detect when an individual needs help or when the process needs to be redesigned

4. Rules of conduct that are aligned with the organization's practical values

5. Expectations for improvement

6. Organizational relationships (external and internal)

■ EXHIBIT 10.2: ROLE DESCRIPTION TEMPLATE

Role Description Template

Role Statement

Position Title: _____

Department Title: _____ Function: _____ Supervisor:

Title: _____

Pay range:	Type of position:	Hours/week: _____
_____ (Depending upon experience and level of responsibility and market)	☐ **Full-time** ☐ **Part-time** ☐ **Temp employee/Contractor** ☐ **Intern**	☐ **Exempt** ☐ **Nonexempt**

OCHIN recognizes that people do their best work and are most satisfied when working in a healthy work environment. OCHIN seeks to nurture a healthy and productive work atmosphere that supports current members of the team and one that is eager to welcome and adapt to new members as they are added. The following values have been identified as essential characteristics and behaviors of OCHIN's work environment. They establish a framework for employee and organizational expectations about what it means to work at OCHIN.

Organization Mission

OCHIN partners with communities to create the knowledge and information solutions to promote access to high-quality and affordable health care for all.

Role Statement—How This Position Supports the Mission

The _____ (role name) supports the mission of OCHIN by

Process and Measurement Responsibilities

All work is a process. Each role has process responsibilities which are interdependent and impact the OCHIN system and network. Processes currently defined for this role have been defined below. We must be alert to defining new processes and eliminating obsolete processes as needs of our role dictate. Performance measurement measures the system and the individual together. Below are the key processes for this role and measures that have been currently defined for this position which will be presented on control charts with a weekly frequency:

Process Name (#)	Process Measurement

Secondary Process Responsibilities (Back Up for Others)

Conduct

The _____ (role name) will model behaviors consistent with the published values of OCHIN.

Responsibilities for Improving the System

All OCHIN employees are responsible for working together to improve the OCHIN network (internally and externally.) Friday afternoons are allocated for this purpose. When changes are considered, we will use the following questions from the Model for Improvement routinely:

What changes do we want to test?

What are we trying to accomplish or learn from these changes?

How will we know a change is an improvement?

(Use of measures will help us understand if our changes are improvements.)

The _____ (role name) is responsible for

- Documenting, communicating, sharing information and developing solutions.
- PDSA cycles are the approach to all improvement work that we undertake.
- Routinely monitoring all personal measures. Special causes will be noted, researched, documented, and action taken, if reasonable. Unacceptable system performance will be submitted for improvement projects. Time will be allocated for improvements that focus on OCHIN or member productivity, improved satisfaction, and elimination of waste.
- Troubleshooting problems independently without escalation whenever possible.
- Knowing how to find answers to questions and ask for help, when appropriate.
- Learning from mistakes and unintended consequences.
- Documenting, communicating, and suggesting solutions for
  - Equipment that needs repair or replacement
  - Things that go wrong and can be prevented
  - Things that could be made easier or more efficient
  - Equipment or supplies that are needed
  - Items identified as a problem or observation
  - Safety incidents or issues
- What does management need to do to make your job better and easier?

Organization Relationships

- The _____ (role) directly reports to _____ and is part of the _____ team.
- The _____ (role) shares information within the OCHIN organization.

External Relationships

Personal Improvement

OCHIN provides $2,500 per year to employees in support for education and training outside the organization. It is the associate's responsibility to seek approval, schedule, and participate in education or training that will prepare him or her for present and future needs.

QUALIFICATIONS/ABILITIES:

_____
_____
_____
_____

Using and Developing Practical Values to Guide Decisions

In 2010, the leadership group developed and published the following practical values for present and future employees. These values permeate decision making as new potential candidates are considered for employment or current associates are coached and developed. Candidates and associates are challenged to verbalize actions in contrast with their values. Contradictions are acknowledged and questioned to ensure alignment for the present and future. Currently these practical values are displayed prominently on the wall of the main staircase at the entrance of the building as a reminder to their importance. Table 10.3 describes these practical values from the perspective of the individual and the OCHIN system.

Initially, some members of the executive team believed that taking the time to define values was a waste of time. However, within the first month of publishing these values, practical applications were evident. When the values were published, all associates felt able to challenge behaviors and decisions which seemed to be in conflict with the stated values. Issues were surfaced and resolved, using the values as the guide. Routinely, executives discuss how to model these values and take action when anyone in

Table 10.3 OCHIN Practical Values for the Individual and System

Practical Values	Individual	The System
Excellence Quality Results and Service Delivery	Critical thinker who is able to make appropriate decisions and find solutions for each situation. Works effectively under pressure meeting deadlines and delivering superior results. Keeps the focus of the customers and striving to meet their needs at the forefront of his work.	The pursuit of creating value which is defined as: Value = Quality/Total Cost
Innovation Future Oriented	Generates new and creative ideas that shape new processes, cuts costs, and improves the overall system that we are working in.	OCHIN encourages creative ideas that promote organizational and individual learning.
Leadership Strategic	Demonstrates vision, courage, respect, and accountability. A leader is one who has followers.	The OCHIN employees are responsible for ensuring constancy of purpose by providing: The will to embrace change, ideas to better serve the purpose, execution of needed changes, and support of the people that make it happen.
Inclusive Engenders Diversity and Learning	Thoughtfully considers and incorporates the diversity of ideas of people and customers in daily decision making through honest and productive communications.	OCHIN recognizes the complexity of our environ-ment and actively seeks out and respects the internal and external input that contrib-utes to our purpose.
Collaboration Teamwork Cooperation Unity	Solves problems and works as a team player to meet member and organizational needs. Makes an effort to find solutions that fit for everyone involved. Understands the value of give and take and looks for strengths in others in order to build productive partnerships.	The OCHIN system thrives when talented and skilled people work together to meet our purpose. OCHIN creates a high value for the organizations it works with and partnerships it builds.

Table 10.3   Continued

Stewardship Service Integrity	Nurtures a fiduciary responsibility to use the money in a conscientious manner. Has a passion for supporting and bettering the environments and communities in which they work. Exhibits trust and honesty.	Everyone striving to make better use of our funds.

the organization's actions is not consistent with them. Analysis of past relationship failures have led OCHIN to now recognize value differences which were not evident before. As future members and partners are considered, their stated values are also reviewed to ensure that OCHIN is the right match.

As a result, values are acknowledged by all executives as a crucial component for OCHIN's success as a learning organization. No longer is the focus just on skills and knowledge; rather, individuals' values are their foundation for decisions. Alignment of individual or organizational values is essential in the execution of OCHIN's collaborative learning environment.

Partnering with Members to Create a Collaborative Structure

When creating a collaborative environment, a primary challenge is to develop a structure where multiple, independent entities share, learn, and cooperate. Such an environment requires prioritization and decision making that cannot focus on one member's needs more than any other. Decisions must be good for the entire system to ensure that OCHIN and the membership benefit. The collaborative has three primary elements:

- A hosted electronic health records and practice management system
- Networking and mentoring (among members)
- Collaboration through shared direction setting and decision making

Elements of the collaborative structure can be seen in Figure 10.17.

Figure 10.17 Member Collaboration Structure

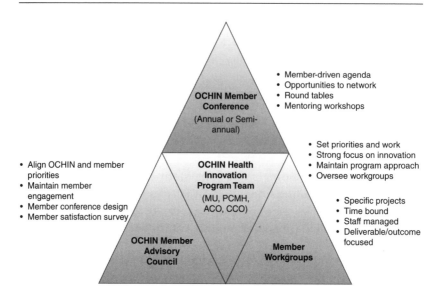

The OCHIN Health Innovation Program Team is the core of the collaborative structure and integrates directly with the OCHIN delivery system and members to charter workgroups with specific 90- to 180-day assignments. This overall structure not only gives members a voice in the collaborative network but also integrates them into the overall delivery system.

Partnering with Members to Transform Health Care

A primary goal of OCHIN is to partner with members and share learning among members. As the data host for the electronic health records for independent clinics and county health departments OCHIN leadership believed this was an operational necessity. Members work collaboratively on clinical readiness, workflow redesign, provider and staff training, hosting, implementation, optimization, reporting, billing, and effective use of practice management and electronic health record (EHR) systems required to achieve strategic clinical, operational, and financial goals. Members also share software data interfaces and capabilities which minimizes the cost to each member to use and update the system.

In 2009 OCHIN sponsored and received a small grant for five members with fifteen community clinics to improve diabetic patient outcomes for their community health in a three-year period from HRSA in the U.S. Department of Health and Human Services. The collaborative[7] agreed to the following three measures as a preliminary step in the application for the grant:

1. Percentage of patients diagnosed with diabetes with the last HbA1c reading done within the last 6 months (see Figure 10.18)

2. Percentage of patients diagnosed with diabetes with the last HbA1c reading <=8 months (see Figure 10.19)

3. Percentage of patients diagnosed with diabetes with depression screening within the last 12 months (see Figure 10.20)

Starting in September 2009, members worked collaboratively on clinical readiness, workflow redesign, receiving provider and staff training in workflow redesign, quality improvement methods, variation, and personality intelligence. They used the data services program called Solutions to manage the patient care and results. The first year, they worked with one clinic in each organization. By the second year, they had spread the improvements to all fifteen clinics with the following results, one year ahead of schedule. OCHIN was recognized by HRSA for achieving the following results in record time.

Figure 10.18   Percent of Patients Diagnosed with DM with HbA1c Done Within 6 Months

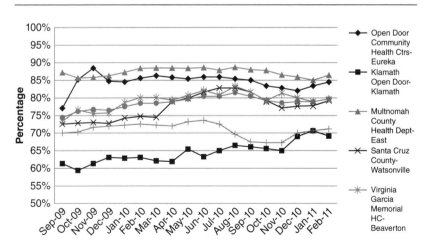

Figure 10.19 Percent of Patients Diagnosed with DM Last HbA1c Reading <=8 Months

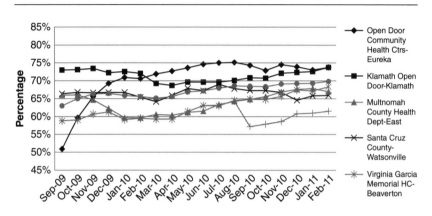

Figure 10.20 Percent of Adult Patients Diagnosed with Diabetes and Screened for Depression Within the Last 12 Months

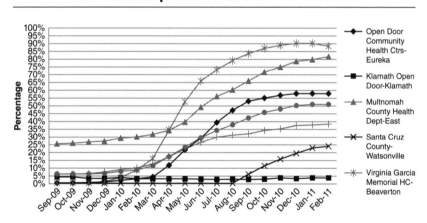

Developing Partners—Outside of OCHIN and Its Members

OCHIN recognizes the value of partnering with not only members, but with private, nonprofit, state and federal government entities in order to achieve its purpose and deliver the best value products and services to its membership. Partnerships require foresight, tenacity, willingness, and creativity to develop relationships that will benefit both parties. Following are some examples where OCHIN has reached beyond their organization's capacity and expertise to provide additional services and products through partnerships:

Products:

- Mid Rogue eHealth Services (MReHS) and OCHIN/O-HITEC announced a partnership that will advance electronic health record adoption in the state of Oregon. MReHS was founded by physicians to promote health care quality, access, and efficiency through the effective use of information technology. They currently provide a hosted implementation of Greenway's PrimeSuite electronic health record (EHR). O-HITEC chose Mid Rogue eHealth Services as a statewide partner to implement Greenways PrimeSuite EHR because of their solid reputation as a Greenway provider in Southern Oregon.

Services:

- EasyStreet® Online Services Inc. as its data center colocation partner.
- Oregon Medical Association to conduct workshop series called "Passport to Health IT." The series is designed specifically for small and medium-sized clinics operating both with and without an EHR. The courses are intended to complement the HITECH programs, language, and organizations in Oregon.
- ORHQN to assist Oregon's twenty-five Critical Access Hospitals in reaching the federal requirement to meaningfully use an electronic health record (EHR).
- Gateway EDI, a leading health care solutions provider of electronic data interchange services to help OCHIN/OHITEC members save time and money.

Summary

In the twelve years of OCHIN's existence, the last two have proven to be the most challenging. Transforming OCHIN from primarily an electronic health record installation company to a health information and technology provider and almost tripling personnel in two years is a likely formula for failure. Yet using the elements of leadership, Sears embarked on this learning journey, building an executive leadership team that was not afraid to learn and grow.

Her vision pushed the bounds of their collective leadership knowledge and experience.

Responding to unexpected consequences and weaknesses in the system required tenacity, trust in the vision, and methods explained in this book. But the benefits have far exceeded the pain along the way, and the bridge is getting stronger every day through collaborative learning from internal talent, member contributions, and outside partnerships. Of course, no one is satisfied and the work goes on to attain better patient health, better community health, and lower costs for health care.

KEY TERMS

Albumin

Building a system of improvement

Chain reaction

County council

EHR

ESRD

OCHIN

Profound knowledge

Project charter

Quality as a Business Strategy (QBS)

Qulturum

Strategic intelligence

ENDNOTES

1. The authors are indebted to Mats Bojestig, Göran Henriks, Abby Sears, and Jerry Jackson for their tireless dedication to learning and improvement, and guidance as we were developing these three case studies.

2. A county council, or *landsting*, is an elected assembly of a county in Sweden. It is a political entity, elected by the county electorate, and its main responsibilities typically are within the public health care system. In each county there is also a county administrative board which is an administrative entity appointed by the government.

3. Gerald J. Langley, Ronald D. Moen, Kevin M. Nolan, Thomas W. Nolan, Clifford L. Norman, and Lloyd P. Provost, *The Improvement Guide: A Practical Approach to Enhancing Organizational Performance*, 2nd ed. (San Francisco: Jossey-Bass, 2009), Figure 13.2.

4. The Institute for Healthcare Improvement (IHI), an independent not-for-profit organization based in Cambridge, Massachusetts, focuses on motivating and building the will for change; identifying and testing new models of care in partnership with both patients and health care professionals; and ensuring the broadest possible adoption of best practices and effective innovations. http://www.ihi.org (accessed June 28, 2012).

5. W. E. Deming, *The New Economics for Industry, Government Education* (Cambridge: MIT, 1993), 93.

6. The clinics included in the case for Dr. Jackson are located in Birmingham, Alabama, and are part of Fresenius Medical Care North America. Fresenius is a major provider of kidney dialysis services and renal care products. Fresenius provides products, dialysis care services, education, and support for chronic kidney disease (CKD), including treatment options for later-stage CKD. http://www.fmcna.com/fmcna/index.htm (accessed June 28, 2012).

7. The clinics included in the OCHIN HRSA grant are located in the state of Oregon and are all clinics which target the medically underserved.

LEADING CHANGE

First Steps in Employing Strategic Intelligence to Get Results

Previous chapters have described the knowledge, methods, tools and qualities of mind and heart needed to lead change. This chapter suggests ways to begin the process of developing an organization and individual leaders for a learning organization through the application of these methods and tools. Table 11.1 gives an overview of twenty-six exercises that may be applicable to you and your leadership team.

Table 11.1 Summary of Exercises for Leading Change

Section	Exercise #
Assessing and Defining Purpose of the Organization	11.1: Questions for the Organization's Executive Leadership
Assessing the Learning Organization	11.2: Learning Organization Evaluation
Aligning Roles to Support the Organization's Purpose	11.3: Develop an Internal Team or Department Role Statement
	11.4: Develop an Individual Role Statement
	11.5: Develop a Role Description
Leading Health Care	11.6: Individual Leadership Responsibilities
Developing a Leadership Philosophy and Practical Values	11.7: Individual Leadership Philosophy
	11.8: Team Leadership Philosophy

(*continued*)

Table 11.1   Continued

Summarizing and Interpreting Results from Practical Values Gap Survey for Leadership Team Learning	11.9: Practical Values Gap Analysis
Strategic Intelligence and Profound Knowledge for Changing Systems	11.10: Individual Strategic Intelligence Inventory
Developing Personality Intelligence	11.11: Individual Personality Intelligence 11.12: Individual Motivation 11.13: Team Motivation
Systems Thinking: Creating a Systems Map of Your Organization	11.14: Map Strategic Objectives to the System Map to Identify Projects 11.15: Utilize the System Map to Consider System Contributions to Problem
Process of Change: Idealized Design	11.16: Using the Four Ps to Create the Idealized Design
Understanding the Psychology of Partners and Collaborators	11.17: Assess Ideal Future Leadership Support 11.18: Assess Ideal Future Organizational Support
Translating the Vision and Strategy to Actionable Approaches	11.19: Strategic Planning Assessment
Leading Individual and Team Improvement Efforts to Achieve the Vision	11.20: Develop a Driver Diagram 11.21: Develop an Ami™ Draft Project Charter from the Driver Diagram
The Sponsor Report: Keeping Leaders in the Communication Loop	11.22: Create a Sponsor Report
Leaders Learning from Improvement Efforts	11.23: Review Projects Using PDSA
Redeployment of Resources	11.24: Resource Allocation
Removing Barriers and Obstacles	11.25: Conduct Improvement Team Review Meeting 11.26: Learning Organization Evaluation

Assessing and Defining Purpose for the Organization

Chapters 2 and 10 describe learning organizations. All are engaged in continuous improvement, some with the Triple Aim of improved patient cases, reduced costs, and a healthy community. Defining purpose is essential for orienting the leaders and staff of your organization. Values and processes should further the purpose. Often done quickly, or soon forgotten, the statement of purpose requires serious thought and continued attention.

The purpose of the organization is the reason the organization exists, the need it fulfills in society. Before writing a statement of purpose, your team should know whether there is a statement of purpose already written elsewhere in the organization that can be used for every part of the organization. If there is, then your team should build on that statement. If no other purpose document exists or the organizational purpose should be modified, then you should discuss the following questions with your team to educate them about their future leadership role:

- What is the purpose of our organization?
- Do we agree to develop a statement of purpose?
- How much time is required?
- Do we agree to discuss and examine our purpose and the vision of how our organization will achieve that purpose?

As the team answers these questions, it becomes ready to define the purpose, and later the organizational vision necessary to achieve it. However, it is useful to understand reasons for dissenting views. This can bring insight to organizational policies, procedures, or traditional behaviors which are in direct conflict with the learning organization, Before the team begins to define a purpose, give everyone present a chance to write out answers to the following questions, and then read them to the team. This can bring out important differences so that people don't go along with an earlier speaker's statement because they want to avoid conflict. By answering the questions in the exercise, the team will become ready to develop the wording to express your purpose in meeting the needs of those you serve. Review the draft of the purpose statement and discuss ways to make it clear and meaningful.

The first draft may include many ideas, and likely be too long and complex. With more work your team can make the draft shorter, with each word taking on more communication power. Consider Abraham Lincoln who made more than a dozen drafts of the Gettysburg Address. Though only a paragraph long, it is considered one of the finest expressions of American literature.

■ STATEMENT OF PURPOSE EXAMPLE

Johnson & Johnson

"The fundamental objective of Johnson & Johnson is to provide scientifically sound, high quality products and services to help heal, cure disease and improve the quality of life."

Cincinnati Children's Hospital

"Cincinnati Children's will improve child health and transform delivery of care through fully integrated, globally recognized research, education and innovation.

"For patients from our community, the nation and the world, the care we provide will achieve the best:

- Medical and quality of life outcomes
- Patient and family experiences and
- Value today and in the future"

Note that these statements describe how the organization will serve its customers or patients. These statements focus the organization on who their customers are, what their customers need and how they differentiate themselves to create value. In contrast, statements like, "Becoming the best in the world," or "Being recognized as a global leader" are too general and don't differentiate the organization's strength or approach (the how we meet the needs) from others. Broad statements do not inspire nor create followers of the idealized vision for the organization.

EXERCISE 11.1
QUESTIONS FOR THE ORGANIZATION'S EXECUTIVE LEADERSHIP

1. What is your organization like now and what do you think it should become?
2. What are the organization's strategic goals?
3. What are reasons for initiating change?
4. What general "need" does the organization fulfill; in other words, why is this organization needed?

5. If a purpose or mission exists, assess it using the questions below:

   a. What needs are we fulfilling in society today and in the future?

   b. Who are our patients or customers?

   c. Why do our patients or customers come to us, rather than elsewhere?

   d. By what methods (major processes, products, and services) do we match their needs?

   e. What is unique about our organization?

   f. Does the current purpose of the organization answer these questions? If not, consider revising the purpose.

6. If a purpose does *not* exist, draft one using the examples above and answering these questions:

   a. What needs are we fulfilling in society today and in the future?

   b. Who are our patients or customers?

   c. Why do our patients or customers come to us, rather than elsewhere?

   d. By what methods do we match their needs?

   e. What is unique about our organization?

Assessing the Learning Organization

EXERCISE 11.2

LEARNING ORGANIZATION EVALUATION

Evaluate your organization (team or business unit) against the attributes of a learning organization.

1. What evidence demonstrates that all employees understand how all the parts of the system interact to achieve the purpose of serving patients?

2. What processes have been designed and redesigned within the system within the past year? Describe the results.

3. What processes are in the process of being designed and redesigned within the system? How were they identified and selected?

4. How is the learning from the change efforts managed? Where does the information reside?

5. How does the organization partner to share changes and learning with stakeholders throughout the system?

6. How does the organization partner with suppliers, client organizations, and community organizations?

7. How do health care professionals routinely collaborate across disciplines, with patients and their families? Describe what has been learned from these interactions and relationships.

8. How do we share learning to inform the community, aid in the prevention of illness, and improve population health?

9. How much time is allocated to improvement and learning for individuals within the system?

10. What changes would you propose to reinforce learning throughout the organization?

Aligning Roles to Support the Organization's Purpose

There should be only one purpose or mission for the organization. In support of the purpose role statements should be articulated. The use of the words *purpose* or *mission* should be reserved for the organization. By utilizing the term *role* for individuals, there is no confusion as to which purpose or mission is most important. Role descriptions do not compete with the purpose; rather they define the intent of the role in a learning organization. In contrast, a job description is a traditional description of compensation, reporting structure, and skills, usually without reference to the organizational system. Role descriptions not only include the traditional information from the job description, but also include responsibility for processes, measures, expected conduct in relation to values, responsibilities for learning, and system improvement. In other words, how the role supports and helps achieve the purpose of the organization.

Role statements should be nested or complementary. Much like Russian nested dolls, the individual role statement should fit inside the organizational team in which it resides. The team's role includes the processes of the individuals and how they nest into the purpose. This provides alignment for the organizational system and helps individuals and teams understand their contributions and responsibilities to the organizational purpose.

As with the purpose statement, the first draft of role descriptions may include many ideas, and likely be too long and complex. Work with the team to make the draft concise, with each word taking on more communication power. Following are some examples to consider.

■ ROLE STATEMENT EXAMPLES

Team/Business Unit

The EPIC operation team supports the mission of OCHIN by efficiently and effectively bringing new members into the collaborative while providing value through ongoing support and service to existing members. We do this by providing high-quality, timely installations, interfaces, and improved platforms through creative and usable solutions to meet the changing needs of members and their patients.

OCHIN Billing Services provides high-value services by efficiently maximizing reimbursement and patient collections, partnering with our members to share innovative and responsible billing practices, and treating their patients with respect and dignity.

Individual

The director for operational excellence directly supports the mission by managing the execution of the quality improvement plan and collaborative initiatives through the development of internal resources for both payers and providers. The manager will define, lead, and support improvement efforts within the payer system through the learning center, which includes assisting and providing resources to providers.

The administration intern supports the Purpose of Profound Knowledge Products, Inc., by preparing high-quality, up-to-date educational and training materials for publication, creating, documenting and updating operational procedures, uploading relevant documents and managing the LMS Cloud, organizing and maintaining the main office documents, files and facilities, identifying and purchasing supplies, while supporting clients and suppliers as needed.

EXERCISE 11.3

DEVELOP AN INTERNAL TEAM OR DEPARTMENT ROLE STATEMENT

a. What needs are we fulfilling for the organization today and in the future?

b. Who are our internal and external customers?

c. Why do our internal and external customers come to us, rather than contract elsewhere?

d. By what methods (processes, products, or services) do we fulfill our internal and external customer's needs?

EXERCISE 11.4

DEVELOP AN INDIVIDUAL ROLE STATEMENT

---

a. What needs does this role fulfill to the organization today and in the future?

b. Who are the internal and external customers?

c. Why do our internal and external customers need this role internally, rather than contract elsewhere?

d. By what methods (processes, products, or services) does this role fulfill their internal and external customer's needs?

EXERCISE 11.5

DEVELOP A ROLE DESCRIPTION

Use the following role description template to develop an example of a complete role description for an individual.

EXHIBIT 11.1   ROLE DESCRIPTION TEMPLATE

Role Description

Position Title:
Department Title:
Function:
Supervisor Title:

Pay Range: (Depending Upon Experience and Level of Responsibility and Market)	Type of position: ☐ Full-time ☐ Part-time ☐ Temp Employee/Contractor ☐ Intern	Hours/week: _____ ☐ Exempt ☐ Nonexempt

Section 1.01: Organization Purpose or Mission

[Insert Organization's Purpose]

Role statement—How this position supports the purpose

The [role] supports the purpose of [organization name] by

Process and Measurement Responsibilities

All work is a process. Each role has process responsibilities which are interdependent and have an impact on [organization name]. Processes currently defined for this role have been defined below. We must be alert to defining new processes and eliminating obsolete processes as needs of our role dictate. Performance measurement analyzes the system and the individual together. Following are the key processes for this role and the measures that have been currently defined for this position which will be presented on control charts with a weekly frequency:

Process Name (#)	Process Measurement

Secondary Process Responsibilities (Backup for Others)

Conduct

The [role name] will model behaviors consistent with the published values of [organization].

Responsibilities for Improving the System

All employees are responsible for working together to improve the [name of the organization] system (internally and externally). When changes are considered, we will use the following questions from the Model for Improvement routinely:

1. What changes do we want to test?

2. What are we trying to accomplish or learn from these changes?

3. How will we know a change is an improvement?

(Use of measures will help us understand if our changes are improvements.)

The [role name] is responsible for

- Documenting, communicating, sharing information, and developing solutions
- PDSA cycles are the approach to all improvement work that we undertake.
- Routinely monitoring all personal measures. Special causes will be noted, researched, documented, and action taken, if reasonable. Unacceptable system performance will be submitted for improvement projects. Time will be prioritized and allocated for improvements that focus on productivity, improved satisfaction, and elimination of waste.
- Troubleshooting problems independently without escalation whenever possible.
- Know how to find answers to questions and ask for help, when appropriate.
- Learn from mistakes and unintended consequences.
- Documenting, communicating, and suggesting solutions for
  - Equipment that needs repair or replacement
  - Things that go wrong and can be prevented
  - Things that could be made easier or more efficient
  - Equipment or supplies that are needed
  - Items identified as a problem or observation
  - Safety incidents or issues
- What does management need to do to make your job better and easier?

Organization Relationships:

- The [role] directly reports to ___ and is part of the ___ team.
- The [role] shares information to [describe what part of the organization].

External Relationships:

Personal Improvement:

Qualifications/Abilities:

_____

_____

_____

_____

Leading Health Care

INDIVIDUAL LEADERSHIP RESPONSIBILITIES

As an individual define your leadership responsibilities, both in the formal organization chart and in informal relationships, by completing the questions below:

1. What is your leadership style?
2. What are your strengths?
3. How do you motivate people to collaborate to achieve the organization's purpose?
4. How successful are you in motivating others? Based on the Five Rs of motivation, what could you change to improve your results?
5. Who are your partners who complement your strengths?
6. What other partners do you need to complement your strengths?
7. Where is leadership needed in the organization?
8. Where are the leadership gaps?
9. What are you doing to influence or fill these gaps?
10. What additional things could be done to fill the leadership gaps?

Developing a Leadership Philosophy
and Practical Values

Developing a personal leadership philosophy reinforces purpose and values, and the way to achieve them. This builds trust when actions model the values articulated and because you have made clear what you stand for.

EXERCISE 11.7

INDIVIDUAL LEADERSHIP PHILOSOPHY

As an individual, write your leadership philosophy:

1. What is your role as a leader?

2. How does that support the purpose of your organization?

3. At what level of ethics and moral reasoning do you want to operate as a leader? Provide some examples of operating at this level.

4. What are the practical values that support your role?

5. How do you define results for your organization?

EXERCISE 11.8

TEAM LEADERSHIP PHILOSOPHY

As a team, write your leadership philosophy:

1. How would you describe your organization's leadership philosophy?

2. Is there a fit with each individual's personal philosophy?

3. Describe practical values essential to achieving that purpose, including ethics and moral reasoning.

4. Compare this list with the organizations published values, if any.

5. Insert all practical values from 3 and 4 (without duplication) into the template below.

   a. Discuss what these values mean.

   b. As individuals, assess each value using Table 11.2.

Table 11.2   Gap Survey Form

Practical Values	Importance	How Well Practiced?	Gap
	1=Not Very Important; 5=Very Important	1=Not Practiced; 5=Practiced Very Well	
1	1 2 3 4 5	1 2 3 4 5	
2	1 2 3 4 5	1 2 3 4 5	
3	1 2 3 4 5	1 2 3 4 5	
4	1 2 3 4 5	1 2 3 4 5	
5	1 2 3 4 5	1 2 3 4 5	
6	1 2 3 4 5	1 2 3 4 5	
7	1 2 3 4 5	1 2 3 4 5	
8	1 2 3 4 5	1 2 3 4 5	
9	1 2 3 4 5	1 2 3 4 5	
10	1 2 3 4 5	1 2 3 4 5	

6. Summarize and discuss results:

   a. How well do the team members agree that these values are important in achieving the organization's purpose?

   b. Evaluate and come up with an agreed-upon list.

7. How well are they being practiced?

8. Use Table 11.3 to document and answer these questions.

   a. Where are the largest gaps?

      1. Document the range of gap from the individual results.

   b. How do we know there is a gap?

      1. Document the evidence in the table.

   c. How can these be closed?

      1. Document ideas to close the gap for each value.

Table 11.3   Value Gap Evidence/Action

Value Description	Value Gap Average/Range	Evidence to Support the Gap Rating	Actions Required to Close the Gap or Keep Alignment

9. Using Table 11.4, document and answer these questions
   a. Using the results from Table 11.3, identify those values with the most alignment using the scores for Most Important.
   b. Document evidence to support the rating.
   c. What structure needs to be in place to support and reinforce these values?

Table 11.4　Aligned Values Evidence/Action

Value	Most Important Avg/Range	Evidence to Support the Alignment Rating	Actions Required to Keep Alignment
1			
2			
etc.			

10. Use Table 11.5 to answer these questions.
    a. How will results be described and measured?
    b. What structure needs to be in place to monitor these results?

Table 11.5　Results Discussion

Value	Result	Description or Metric and Frequency of Measurement
1	1	
2	2	
etc.	etc.	

Summarizing and Interpreting Results from the Practical Values Gap Survey for Leadership Team Learning

In Chapter 4 we discussed surveying leaders on how they would rate the stated values of the organization in terms of importance and how well the values are practiced. The leaders who took the Strategic Intelligence Inventory also took the gap survey. They rated six values:

- Excellence
- Innovation
- Leadership

- Inclusivity
- Collaboration
- Stewardship

The gap analysis showed that two values were rated low in performance; excellence and stewardship (see Figure 11.1). A discussion ensued about excellence; many leaders thought they should do everything for a customer no matter the cost. They prided the organization as putting quality first without regard to cost. They liked the reputation of being the Nordstrom's of their industry. The CEO then jotted some notes on the overhead and noted the relationship between stewardship and excellence. She noted that a better word would be providing "value" for customers, value being defined as Value = Quality/Total Cost. "As good stewards," she said "we need to make sure we deliver value, but as leaders we also have to be conscious about the cost of delivering because this can drive up prices in the future for our customers." The team found the discussion useful in defining their roles as leaders in

Figure 11.1   Example of Value Gap Analysis Results

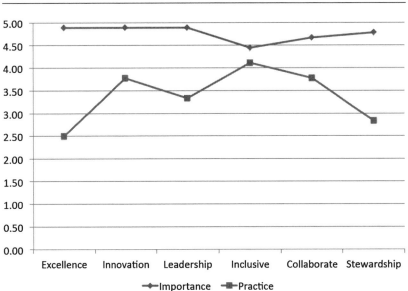

the stewardship of scarce resources. "Excellence" was changed to "Value" with the definition added.

Graphical analysis of the output from both the Strategic Intelligence Inventory and the gap survey on practical values helped to facilitate a useful discussion for the leaders. The charts gave each leader an idea of how they answered relative to their colleagues. They were also able to use the theory of variation and control charts to gain more insight into their answers and their organization.

EXERCISE 11.9

PRACTICAL VALUES GAP ANALYSIS

Graph the practical values gap for your organization's values.

1. What practical values show the least importance? Why?

2. What practical values have the greatest gaps and pose the greatest challenges? Why?

3. Should the practical values be revised based on what was learned?

4. What could be done to reduce the gaps?

Strategic Intelligence and Profound Knowledge for Changing Systems

EXERCISE 11.10

INDIVIDUAL STRATEGIC INTELLIGENCE INVENTORY

As an individual score yourself on the Strategic Intelligence Inventory below.

1. What areas of your strategic intelligence show strength?

2. What areas most need developing?

3. What could you do to improve your personal strategic intelligence?

4. Invite some of your colleagues to partner with you in the spirit of joint learning and development.

5. Summarize and discuss the differences. See example following the Inventory.

Table 11.6   Strategic Intelligence Inventory

Foresight

1	I scan the business or professional environment for trends that present threats to and opportunities for my organization.	1 2 3 4 5
2	I seek out and listen to people whose knowledge helps me foresee future trends.	1 2 3 4 5
3	I construct scenarios of possible futures and think about how my team would deal with each scenario.	1 2 3 4 5
4	I talk to customers and suppliers about their needs.	1 2 3 4 5
5	I study organizations that are very successful and unsuccessful.	1 2 3 4 5
6	I look for patterns in my business environment that indicate future trends.	1 2 3 4 5
7	I keep track of leading indicators from employees and customers that suggest future trends.	1 2 3 4 5
8	I look for talented people who can become future leaders.	1 2 3 4 5
9	I study unexpected results, consider their implications, opportunities for the future, and act accordingly.	1 2 3 4 5

Visioning

1	I can describe how my vision uniquely positions my organization in the market.	1 2 3 4 5
2	I can describe how my vision takes account of threats and opportunities for the organization.	1 2 3 4 5
3	I can describe my vision as an idealized design of a social system.	1 2 3 4 5
4	My vision for the organization includes how people will interact with one another.	1 2 3 4 5
5	My vision for the organization includes the practical values essential to its implementation.	1 2 3 4 5
6	I can describe the competencies we need to implement the vision.	1 2 3 4 5
7	My vision includes the design and redesign of processes essential to achieving it.	1 2 3 4 5
8	I incorporate the best ideas of my partners in developing the organizational vision.	1 2 3 4 5
9	My vision includes a plan for its implementation.	1 2 3 4 5

(continued)

Table 11.6 Continued

Systems Thinking

1	I evaluate parts of the organization on how well they further the purpose of the system.	1 2 3 4 5
2	I manage and influence the interactions between different parts of the organization.	1 2 3 4 5
3	When I have a problem, I look for contributing factors before I try to solve it.	1 2 3 4 5
4	When I have several things to do, I try to understand how each action will affect the short- and long-term consequences for the system before I act.	1 2 3 4 5
5	When my theories don't work, I question my assumptions about my understanding of the interdependencies within the system.	1 2 3 4 5
6	I make sure we are developing and hiring people with the competence and values essential to achieve the purpose and vision of the system.	1 2 3 4 5
7	I advocate practical values that further the purpose of the system I lead.	1 2 3 4 5
8	I make sure incentives and rewards strengthen the organizational values and purpose of the system.	1 2 3 4 5
9	I think of my own well-being as an interaction of my physical, mental, and spiritual selves and I work on all three.	1 2 3 4 5

Motivating and Empowering

1	I communicate a philosophy that people in my organization find meaningful.	1 2 3 4 5
2	I affirm people's strengths and place them in roles where they will be motivated.	1 2 3 4 5
3	I do not punish honest mistakes but use them as an opportunity for learning, so that people are not afraid to be open.	1 2 3 4 5
4	I use opposition to reach better solutions.	1 2 3 4 5
5	I am persuasive with resistant colleagues.	1 2 3 4 5
6	I understand the motivating values of the employees who are essential to my organization.	1 2 3 4 5
7	I make sure that our processes and incentives strengthen collaboration.	1 2 3 4 5

Table 11.6   Continued

8	I can tell when people are only paying lip service to the purpose and vision.	1 2 3 4 5
9	I make sure people's contributions are recognized.	1 2 3 4 5
10	People in my organization feel empowered to propose improvements.	1 2 3 4 5

Partnering

1	I know my strengths and seek out partners who complement my strengths.	1 2 3 4 5
2	I know my weaknesses and seek out partners who can help me develop or can compensate for my weaknesses.	1 2 3 4 5
3	I make sure that my partners in the organization share my philosophy of leadership.	1 2 3 4 5
4	I spell out what I expect from partnering.	1 2 3 4 5
5	I seek partners who will tell me hard truths.	1 2 3 4 5
6	I break off ineffective partnering relationships in a timely way.	1 2 3 4 5
7	I partner with key customers to reduce total costs in our joint systems.	1 2 3 4 5
8	I partner with key suppliers to reduce total costs in our joint systems.	1 2 3 4 5
9	I build trust with partners by making sure our philosophies are compatible.	1 2 3 4 5
10	I make sure that my partners will also benefit from our partnerships; relationship are win-win.	1 2 3 4 5

Summarizing and Interpreting Results from the Strategic Intelligence Inventory for Leadership Team Learning

If we have several leaders in the room, how do we display the results of the Strategic Intelligence Inventory so that all can learn about the leadership team's strengths and challenges? As we noted in Chapter 7 on statistical thinking, the graphical display of data makes it easier to understand and gain meaning from the data we collect. The Strategic Intelligence Inventory and Gap Survey Form are no different. One of

Figure 11.2 Strategic Intelligence Survey: Chart Display of Thirty-Eight Questions

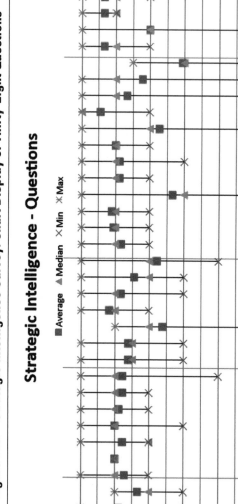

Key: 1-Strongly Disagree, 2-Disagree, 3-Neither Agree nor Disagree, 4-Agree, 5-Strongly Agree

our clients had members of their leadership team take the Strategic Intelligence Inventory and the gap analysis on practical values. One of the authors of this book then took the data and displayed it graphically. Figure 11.2 describes all thirty-eight questions; the questions are grouped by the components of strategic intelligence: foresight, systems thinking, visioning, motivation, and partnering. For each question the high and low scores are depicted for the leadership team. In addition, the average and median scores are also calculated.

From the data in the chart, we can see variation in the way the leadership teams answered certain questions. We can see that responses to the first two groups of questions had less variation than the last three groups of questions. We can see that five of the twelve questions about motivation varied to zero. When the leadership team saw these results, they discussed the meaning of these results. This discussion led to thinking about who on the leadership team should be taking the lead on the various strategic intelligence issues.

These data were examined with the control chart method. For the systems thinking question #1: "I evaluate parts of the organization and its systems in terms of how well they further the overall purpose," the X Bar and S charts (see Figure 11.3) show that the average response for this question was 4.0. The standard deviation for the responses is zero; in other words, high agreement with no variation in response for the team. The group also was in agreement in response to question #6 about evaluating parts of the system to further the overall purpose. But question #30, "Once I know that people are not adding value, I am quick to get rid of them," elicited a low rating of 2.0. The leaders tried to justify the incongruence between these two statements. Eventually, one brave lady stated: "This is a problem for me. I can now see that my reluctance to act on individuals who are not contributing is a problem. I need to work on this issue as a manager."[1]

Responses to question #22, "I understand the values of the investors who are essential to my business," showed outside the limits on both the average and standard deviation. In the discussion that followed, the CEO was able to help the managers understand who the investors were and why they were important to achieving the overall purpose. Once explained, each of the managers said they would now rate the question differently.

The discussion of the questions and how they answered the Strategic Intelligence Inventory led to questions about how the leaders

Figure 11.3 Strategic Intelligence Survey: Control Chart Display (OCHIN)

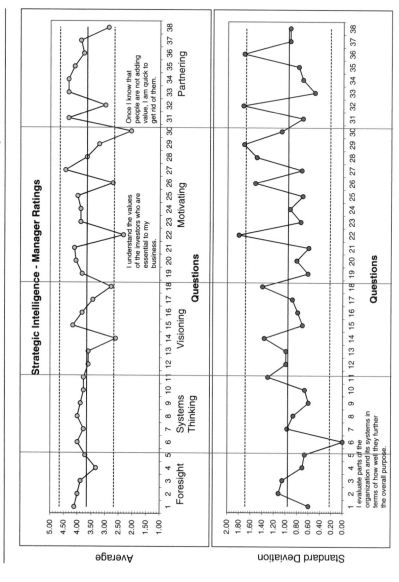

Figure 11.4 Control Chart Organized by Leader

1-Strongly Disagree, 2-Disagree, 3-Neither Agree nor Disagree, 4-Agree, 5-Strongly Agree

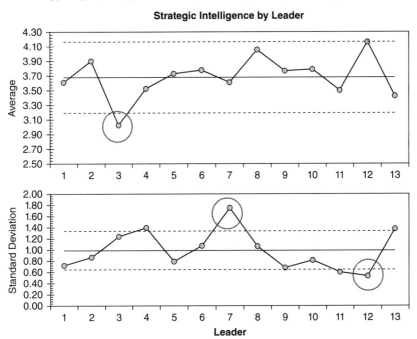

Strategic Intelligence by Leader

answered it individually. Figure 11.4 describes the X Bar and S chart by leader. Leaders 3 and 7 were new to their job and inexperienced which contributed to their low scores, which show as special causes relative to other leaders. Leader 3 has low average for all responses and leader 7 has the most variation in answers versus the other leaders. Leader 12 is a very experienced leader and had the highest average and lowest variation (see special cause circled in Figure 11.4) in responses on all questions.

Developing Personality Intelligence

Understanding yourself and others develops your personality intelligence, and strengthens your ability to inspire and empower others.

```
EXERCISE 11.11
```

INDIVIDUAL PERSONALITY INTELLIGENCE

1. Complete the Leadership Personality Survey found in the Appendix.[2]
2. Complete the Social Character Questionnaire in the Appendix.
3. Read the interpretation of scores in the Appendix for these surveys.

   a. What does this express about your personality that gave you new insight?

   b. How does this drive your approaches to work and relationships?

   c. How does this differ from others with whom you work?

```
EXERCISE 11.12
```

INDIVIDUAL MOTIVATION

As an Individual, describe how you are motivated by the Five Rs.

1. What types of Responsibilities are important to you?
2. What types of Reasons are important to you?
3. What kinds of Relationships are important to you?
4. How do you want to be Recognized?
5. How do you want to be Rewarded?
6. How is this related to your personality?

```
EXERCISE 11.13
```

TEAM MOTIVATION

As a team:

1. As individuals, complete Exercises 14 and 15.
2. Compare the results from each of the Five Rs.
3. Describe how the Rs that motivate you are different or similar to others' motivation.
4. Look at these differences in terms of personality and social character. Remember that each personality type contributes insights and capacities the team needs for success.

5. How do you think differences affect the Five Rs of motivation for you as compared to the others with whom you work?

6. Share experiences where each others' personality types produced conflict, which can be avoided when you are aware of each others' motivations.

   a. How are reasons communicated?

   b. How are responsibilities differentiated and communicated?

   c. How are good relationships maintained?

   d. How do the team members prefer to be recognized?

   e. What type of rewards are important?

7. Ask your colleagues to do those two surveys for themselves.

8. Summarize and compare your scores and answers to question 3.

Systems Thinking: Creating a System Map of Your Organization

The key to systems thinking is to understand that all work is a process and those processes are interconnected. We need everyone to be focused and learning together to reduce the potential for harm and increase our ability to deliver the best possible care to our patients. A learning organization requires a transformation from viewing the organization as a bureaucratic hierarchy of people reporting to each other to a system where the patient (customer) is the focus of the system. The system map (or linkage of processes) is a useful systems thinking tool to help people view the processes within their organizations and how they link together to achieve the purpose. Leaders design, integrate, and align these diverse components so that they serve the purpose of the organization. Ultimately, the success of an organization will depend on this interaction rather than the performance of the individual components.

Figure 11.5 is an example of a macro-level view of the Health Care System initially created with the help of Jönköping County in Sweden with leaders collaborating from Ambulatory Care, Dental Care, Hospital Care, Social Care, Pharmacy and others. The original has been shared, tested and modified for over five years in Canada, Singapore, Britain, Indian Health Services, and locations throughout the United States.

For those who are managing change and creating improvement results, the following Meso System Map (Figure 11.6) for managing

Figure 11.5   Example of a Macro-Level View of the Health Care System

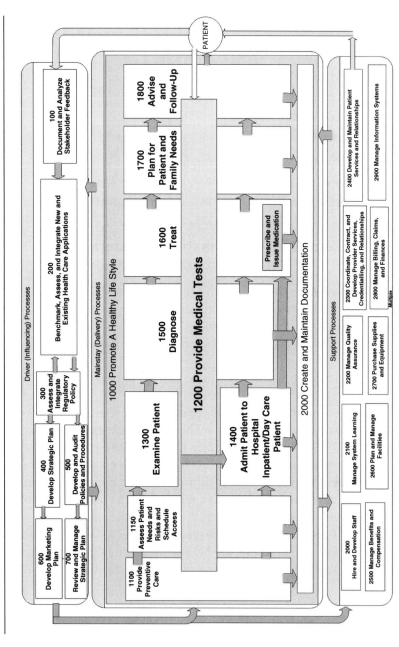

Figure 11.6   Meso System Map for Managing a Learning Organization

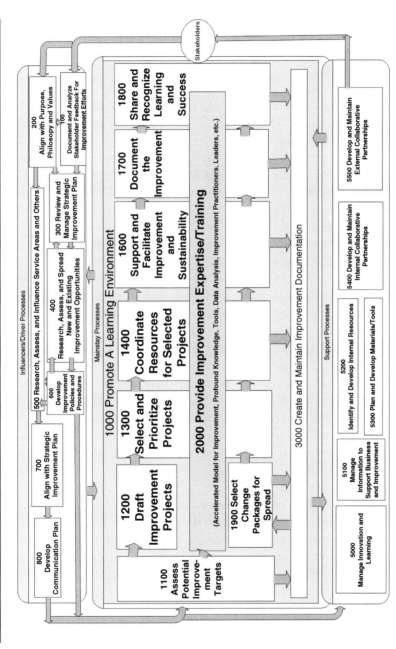

learning within an organization is useful. It has influenced Care Oregon Learning Center in Portland, Oregon, as they developed their capability for improvement. It was developed while running change and improvement in another industry for nine states and Puerto Rico by Jane Norman.

Both examples are conceptual level system maps, one at the macro level and one at the meso level. As all work is a process, you will notice that each box *names* the process by describing the *action* that is being taken. A system map is NOT a flow chart. It links processes and shows relationships, whereas a flow chart describes the steps and decisions in the process. Process naming protocol requires that we do NOT use things or nouns. Processes start with action words or verbs. They do not use ambiguous words such as "process the patient"; instead they would use "schedule the patient visit" or "discharge the patient." The level of detail used in the micro level will determine the name of the process which could later be flow-charted, if needed.

Complex processes are routinely grouped and identify related processes that require coordination and integration. Remember, our system has been perfectly designed to get the outcomes we are getting. If we are not satisfied with the outcomes, processes may be missing or the processes within the system need to be standardized or redesigned in order to achieve the purpose of the organization. Defining the links between processes helps define the relationships and the impact that changes can make to other parts of the system. Links relate to handoffs and how one process connects with another. When processes have weak or nonexistent links, the system breaks and problems occur. Transferring useful information between processes is a common flaw in many systems and a critical issue for health care and the patient.

Within health care, as we learned in the dialysis case with Dr. Jackson, the patient must be treated as a system as well. Yet the structure of our system allows medical specialties (dental, renal, heart, and so on) which dissect the patient and can easily diagnose different patient systems independently. The intent of the electronic medical records is to allow all health care professionals to have access to all of the information for a healthy or sick patient to restore or maintain their health. The challenge is to proactively create a system that is integrated with the human system to prevent sick care and promote health.

EXERCISE 11.14

MAP STRATEGIC OBJECTIVES TO THE SYSTEM MAP TO IDENTIFY PROJECTS

1. Using existing strategic objectives for your organization or team:

    a. Identify what processes or groups of processes are related to each objective, identify and add them within the general process group on the health care system map.

    b. Identify what processes will need additional resources.

    c. Identify processes, products, or services that need to be redesigned in order to meet the objectives. Put a circle on the map.

    d. Identify processes, products, or services that are missing and will need to be designed in order to achieve the objectives. Make sure you have added these to the map. Put a star on the map.

    e. Write charters for any processes defining what is to be designed or redesigned and the desired outcome.

EXERCISE 11.15

UTILIZE THE SYSTEM MAP TO CONSIDER SYSTEM CONTRIBUTIONS TO PROBLEM

1. Use the system map to identify source processes for problems and patterns by asking the following questions:

    a. Where was the problem detected?

    b. What process(es) contributed to the problem? Trace on the system map.

        1. What drivers or influencing processes are related to the problem process(es)?

        2. What support processes are related to the problem process(es)?

    c. Would it be easy for this problem to happen again?

    d. How often does this happen?

    e. How much does the system design contribute to this problem versus the individual(s) who work in the process under investigation?

    f. Investigate these processes in person to see other contributing factors.

2. Look for patterns.

3. Identify new processes to design or redesign in order to prevent these processes.

Process of Change: Idealized Design

Drawing on your foresight and what emerges from your discussion with colleagues, what is your view of the threats and opportunities your organization is facing? How should you respond to them? What is your systemic vision of what the organization should become to further its purpose? Objective: What will the organization look like today if it was producing ideal results? This ideal should meet these criteria:

1. It should be technologically feasible.
2. It should have operational viability, meaning the system is capable of surviving if it is brought into existence.
3. It should be capable of rapid learning and adaptation.

How would you create collaboration for effectiveness and learning? For example, if you have a value of collaboration, are employees evaluated and promoted based on their proven capacity to collaborate? In the same sense, if you value partnering, is your administrative staff evaluated on their skill in partnering with suppliers? If you have a value of "putting the patient first," are staff and systems evaluated on fast attention to patient needs? If evaluations are not aligned with values, how will you address this and align them? When you complete the Four P picture of your **ideal future**, you will have a blueprint for what you and your colleagues need to build together. The OCHIN case study is an example of redesigning the organizational system for an idealized design.

EXERCISE 11.16

USING THE FOUR Ps TO CREATE THE IDEALIZED DESIGN

1. Describe your organization as it is today.

    a. What is the current purpose?

    b. What practical values support the purpose?

    c. What are the key processes, products, and services?

    d. What are the current roles and skills required by our people? How well are people being managed and motivated?

    e. What are the measures used to see how well the organization achieves purpose?

2. Describe your organization in the future.

    a. Purpose

       1. What changes will be required in our purpose to describe our vision?

    b. Practical Values

       1. What changes will be required in our practical values to achieve our vision?

    c. Processes, Products, and Services

       1. What processes must be designed or redesigned to accomplish our vision and support the change?

       2. What are the leverage processes (most important) to ensure our success in achieving the vision? Reference your systems map.

       3. What products and services must be designed or redesigned to achieve our vision?

       4. What processes are needed for collaboration and sharing?

       5. What processes are needed for recognition?

    d. People

       1. What are the roles and responsibilities we need to fill and what kinds of people do we need to fill them?

       2. What are the skills they need to have?

       3. How should they interact? What are the important relationships?

       4. What kinds of personality traits are we looking for?

       5. What is meaningful work for them?

       6. What kinds of relationships do we need to manage?

       7. How will work be evaluated and rewarded?

3. Use Table 11.7 to consider your Four Ps today, and one, three, and five years toward your ideal future. Consider Figure 11.7 as you answer these questions and complete the table.

    a. What leadership process will be required to achieve the vision?

    b. What new leadership actions and interactions are needed throughout the organization?

Table 11.7 Four Ps Planning Template for 1, 3, 5 Years

	Today	In One Year	In Three Years	In Five Years
Purpose				
Practical Values				
Processes				
People				

Figure 11.7 Achieving the Vision of an Ideal Future

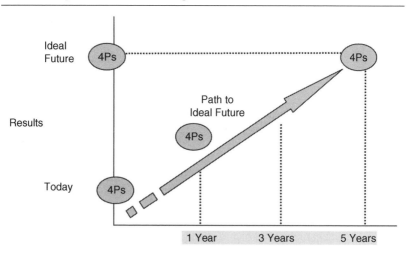

Understanding the Psychology of Partners and Collaborators

Your ability to bring about the ideal future you and your team have just envisioned requires placing people in the right roles (see the OCHIN case in Chapter 10) and leading them in such a way that triggers their intrinsic motivation. Knowing yourself well heightens your ability to know others.

EXERCISE 11.17
ASSESS IDEAL FUTURE LEADERSHIP SUPPORT

Determine how each of your team members is motivated to implement the ideal future you have designed together. Go back to Exercises 11.11–11.13 and complete them.

EXERCISE 11.18

ASSESS IDEAL FUTURE ORGANIZATIONAL SUPPORT

Now that you have described the ideal future of your organization, and what leaders must do to achieve it, you can compare the current organization to the future ideal. Start with a gap survey (Table 11.8) to measure how much others agree with the importance of the elements of the vision (the Four Ps) in achieving the defined purpose.

Table 11.8   Four Ps Gap Survey

Four Ps	Importance	How Well Practiced?	Gap
	1=Not Very Important; 5=Very Important	1=Not Practiced; 5=Practiced Very Well	
Redefined Purpose	1 2 3 4 5	1 2 3 4 5	
Redefined Practical Values	1 2 3 4 5	1 2 3 4 5	
Redefined Processes	1 2 3 4 5	1 2 3 4 5	
Redefined People Skills	1 2 3 4 5	1 2 3 4 5	

1. How well do they see the organization implementing those elements today? You can use the aggregate survey responses to discuss with people throughout the organization what needs to be done to close the gaps.

2. These groups should agree on plans to close the gaps. The groups may need a facilitator at first, although some leaders may be able to facilitate their own groups. Many visionary leaders are not good at getting people to state their ideas openly. And people are often silent out of fear of the leader or their colleagues and instead parrot back what they think the leader wants. Leaders can learn how to facilitate by observing a skilled facilitator. After a period of implementing steps to the ideal, you can assess progress with another gap survey.

Translating the Vision and Strategy to Actionable Approaches

Effective leaders describe a vision and work with others to develop a strategy for implementation.

EXERCISE 11.19

STRATEGIC PLANNING ASSESSMENT

As the leadership team of the organization, how do you accomplish the following in your organization?

1. Identify strategies to accomplish the vision.

2. Ensure that the strategies are carried out.

3. Communicate and coordinate among groups of people across departmental boundaries.

4. Coordinate education and training for individuals and teams.

5. Identify barriers that inhibit continuous improvement and coordinate the removal of these barriers.

6. Manage overlapping responsibilities of individuals and teams.

7. Study the quality improvement efforts to learn about fundamental causes of problems in the organization.

8. Evaluate and publicize the status of the improvement process.

9. Redirect and redeploy resources as improvements are made.

To ensure that these nine tasks are accomplished requires a concerted effort on the part of the leadership team. We will discuss the role of a leader in translating the vision into action. This journey is usually complex and can be made easier by the use of simple tools. Our clients have found it useful to use the following communication and coordination tools:

1. The driver diagram
2. Draft Ami™ Charter
3. Sponsor report

A useful tool in making strategic actions explicit is called a **driver diagram** (see Figure 11.8). The initial driver diagram for a strategy might lay out the descriptive theory (discussed in Chapter 9) of desirable outcomes that can be tested and enhanced to develop a predictive theory. The driver diagram should be updated throughout a change effort and used to track progress in theory building. Figure 11.8 presents a driver diagram for improving clinic access and reducing wait times. This would be a large undertaking with the purpose of achieving the Triple Aim.

Figure 11.8 Driver Diagram for Achieving Improved Patient Experience, Population Health, and Reduced per Capita Cost

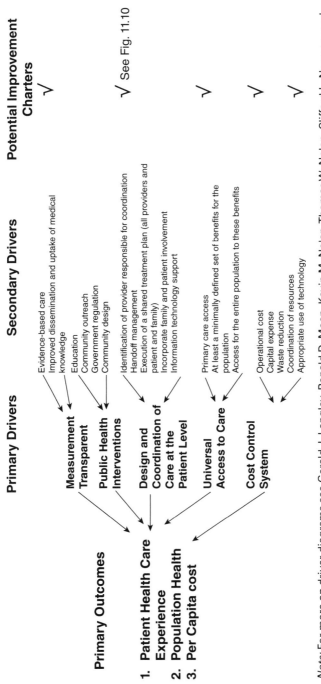

Note: For more on driver diagrams see Gerald J. Langley, Ronald D. Moen, Kevin M. Nolan, Thomas W. Nolan, Clifford L. Norman, and Lloyd P. Provost, *The Improvement Guide: A Practical Approach to Enhancing Organizational Performance*, 2nd ed. (San Francisco: Jossey-Bass, 2009), 429.

Figure 11.9   Driver Diagram Template

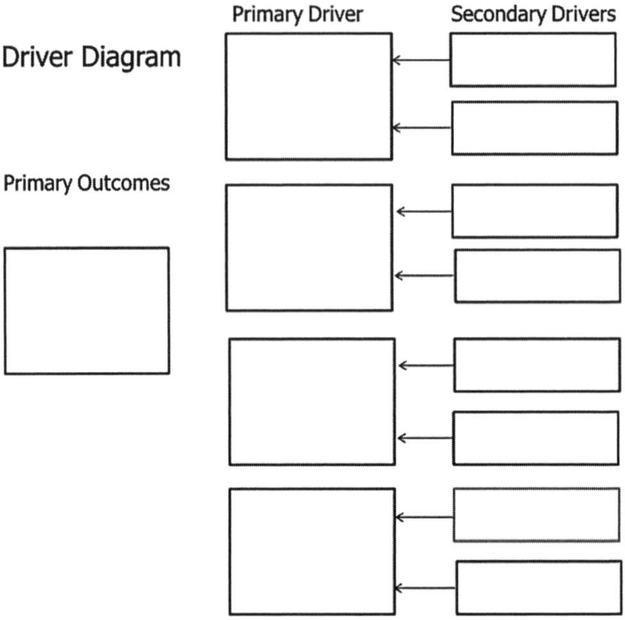

Ideas for change can now be generated from the secondary driver column. These changes will lead to specific improvement projects to accomplish your vision. Figure 11.9 is a blank form for you to sketch out a driver diagram for your strategies to accomplish your vision. The charter example to follow in Figure 11.10 will pick up on the use of this driver diagram with an example.

Leading Individual and Team Improvement Efforts to Achieve the Vision

Leadership should be actively involved in improvement efforts.

EXERCISE 11.20

DEVELOP A DRIVER DIAGRAM

Use the Driver Diagram Template (Figure 11.9) to identify the outcomes that strategically are important to the organization.

The Ami™ is designed to communicate the purpose of a team or individual involved in an improvement effort. One of the primary responsibilities of leaders involved in change is to align the people in the organization with strategic improvement efforts to accomplish the vision. The Model for Improvement (MFI) introduced in Chapter 9, is a useful framework for a project charter. The first two of the three MFI questions should be answered by a leader or by the leadership team:

1. What are we trying to accomplish?
2. How will we know that a change is an improvement?

Without a clear project charter, it is easy to get sidetracked and work in areas of minor relevance to the key initiatives of the organization. The project charter helps teams and individuals manage their efforts and reduce unwanted variations from the original aim as well as know when they have completed their project.

EXERCISE 11.21

DEVELOP AN AMI™ DRAFT PROJECT CHARTER FROM THE DRIVER DIAGRAM

1. Create a draft charter by answering the first two questions on the Ami™ Charter (Figure 11.10).

    a. What will be designed or redesigned in order to achieve the outcomes that strategically are important to the organization.

    b. Identify the current situation and boundaries for the team.

    c. Identify team members based on the process or product which must be designed or redesigned. In the "Secondary Drivers" column note the idea of "Identification of provider responsible for coordination." This will be the sponsor for the team.

    d. From the driver diagram identify the goals that must be accomplished for the project to be completed. Goals for the project with expected results are noted with measures to ensure that the question is answered: How will we know that a change is an improvement?

    e. Figure 11.10 shows the Draft Ami™ Charter that addresses these first two questions.

Figure 11.10   Draft Ami™ Charter

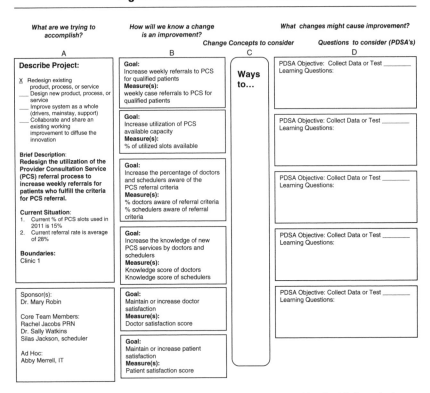

Source: © Profound Knowledge, 2011. All Rights Reserved. Used with Permission.

Using this Ami™ Draft Charter form has proven effective in getting individuals and teams on the right track and minimizing miscommunication between a leader and the people who are making strategic changes to accomplish the vision. Examples of using the model can be found in the cases described in Chapter 10.

The Sponsor Report: Keeping Leaders in the Communication Loop

Once a project is launched, a sponsor from the leadership team should be assigned to the individual or team to ensure that the improvement project stays on track. Leaders from the organization that sponsor project charters for improvement should check the status of teams regularly, by attending meetings or reading status reports. Sponsors should note:

- Achievements of each chartered effort.
- Other departments or individuals not on the team that are providing support.
- Outside resources required for support.
- Teams that are learning, but have not yet made improvements.

Figure 11.11 provides a sample for a **sponsor report** that places this information on one-page for the sponsor. Note the Progress Rating Score in the lower left. The operational definition of these scores can be accessed in Table 11.9.

The decision to designate sponsors for improvement efforts should be made with three considerations in mind:

1. The complexity and formality of the change effort should be evaluated. If the scope is large and involves many people, other organizations, or departments, then a sponsor is usually required.
2. How much authority has been delegated to the team? When informal efforts do not impact others and where teams are aligned to act independently, a sponsor may not be necessary.
3. How complex is the organization in which the improvement effort must be executed? Larger organizations may find sponsors necessary to simplify communication and to ensure that management stays in touch with improvement efforts.

The sponsor is typically a member of the leadership team who will represent the people carrying out the change with other leaders. Sponsors will remove barriers to success and routinely keep other leaders up to date with the progress and issues faced by the change effort. Sponsors are ultimately responsible for the success (or failure) of the team. The sponsor is responsible for

1. Working to reach agreement on the project charter.
2. Providing the resources needed.
3. Assisting the team leader as requested.
4. Keeping the team informed of issues they may need to integrate into the team charter or avoid.

Figure 11.11   Sponsor Report Example: Clinic Wait Time for Patients

Clinic Town Center

Sponsor Report

Reduce laboratory waiting time for patients doing fasting blood test at clinic

Project 7Wave10 Report Date:

Core Team
- Dr. Jane Newton
- Rosa Trevino, RN
- Jon Edwards, RN

What are we trying to accomplish?
Redesign the laboratory scheduling and workflow for patients who are fasting for blood tests at the clinic to reduce wait time

How will we know it is an improvement?
- Reduce laboratory waiting time for patients doing fasting blood test
- Increase patient satisfaction for laboratory services
- Maintain or increase staff satisfaction
- Maintain waiting time for patient doing nonfasting blood test

Evidence Based Improvements and Savings

Progress Rating = 8

Measurement Results (Insert below)
1) Wait time fasting patients
2) Wait time non-fasting patient

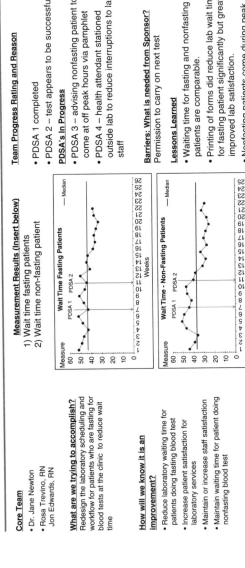

Approved by Project Sponsor

Dr. Daniel Kim...
Name/Signature/Designation/Date

Team Progress Rating and Reason
- PDSA 1 completed
- PDSA 2 – test appears to be successful

PDSA's In Progress
- PDSA 3 – advising nonfasting patient to come at off peak hours via pamphlet
- PDSA 4 – health attendant stationed outside lab to reduce interruptions to lab staff

Barriers: What is needed from Sponsor?
Permission to carry on next test

Lessons Learned
- Waiting time for fasting and nonfasting patients are comparable.
- Printing of forms did reduce lab wait time for fasting patient significantly but greatly improved lab satisfaction.
- Nonfasting patients come during peak hour as they are not aware of opening times. Most are agreeable to come at off peak hour in future.

Recommendations
- Use nonfasting logo from current lab form on pamphlet.

EXERCISE 11.22
CREATE A SPONSOR REPORT

Consider an improvement effort that is currently going on in your organization. Using the sponsor report as an example, have the individual or team complete it for your review.

Learning from Improvement Efforts

The work of improvement teams and other improvement efforts provides leaders an opportunity to learn about the system they are leading. The leadership team should study the work and progress of these improvement activities to learn how the organization works as a system. Learning should include

- **Key processes in the organization and key linkages between processes.** Sometimes when a change is made to a process, there is an unexpected impact in other processes. This learning can be used to update the systems view of the organization to increase systems integration.
- **Underlying forces in the organization that cause problems and create barriers.** What are the management systems (such as accounting, budgeting, appraisal, and so forth) that drive the organization? Study of improvement teams can uncover how these forces interact and impact the employees of the organization.
- **The impact of team improvements on the system.** Often improvement efforts result in cost savings, productivity improvements, and other efficiencies for particular products and particular processes in the organization. How do these improvements affect the key measures of the system (the total organization)? Because the processes and products are not additive, the combined improvements will not add up at the system level. A small improvement at a key part of the system may have a big impact, though it may require many such efforts to make an incremental improvement relative to some other desired outcome.
- **The measured impact of improvements in the system.** How do the various types of improvements result in changes to the care of individual patients? How can this learning be transferred to the larger patient population?

- **The long-term social consequences of technical changes.** How do changes made by improvement teams impact the organization's culture?
- **Understanding the patient's definition of excellent care.** What types of improvements are appreciated by patients and their families?

If you are using a formal leadership meeting to recognize a team, the Model for Improvement can be used to help leaders focus their learning. Each time a meeting is scheduled with an individual or team involved that is presenting an improvement effort, the leaders should plan a Plan-Do-Study-Act (PDSA) cycle. The most important part of the plan will be

- What specific questions do we want to answer?
- What are our predictions about the answers to these questions?

After the team meeting or presentation is completed (the "Do" phase of the cycle), the leaders can evaluate the answers they obtained ("Study") and take appropriate actions ("Act") based on what they have learned.

EXERCISE 11.23
REVIEW PROJECTS USING PDSA

Consider having two or three teams or people present their improvement projects. (This exercise can be combined with 11.25.)

A. *Plan:* Prior to the meeting and as a leadership team, predict and document answers to the following questions. Ensure that the team is given the questions so that they are answered during their presentation.

 1. What is the team trying to accomplish?

 a. What process(es) or services are being targeted for change?

 b. What outcome measure will be positively affected?

 c. What was the current situation before the team began?

 2. How will the team know their changes will be improvements?

 a. What measures will be improved?

 b. What measures are being followed to ensure other processes or services are creating unintended consequences?

 c. How will this effort impact the Triple Aim?

    3. What changes have been tested?

        a. How are these tests documented for present and future learning?

        b. Have these changes affected the measures and goals?

        c. What has been learned?

        d. What barriers need leadership intervention to ensure the project is completed successfully?

        e. Who has helped the team test the changes and learn?

    4. How long has the team been working on this improvement effort?

    5. What is their estimate for completion?

B. *Do:* Meet with the teams documenting actual information presented by the teams. Focus on the questions and learning.

C. *Study:* After the teams leave, take time to discuss what was learned by comparing the leadership predictions with the team report.

    1. Where were there differences?

    2. What new issues were identified?

D. *Act:* Discuss what actions are needed by the leadership team to support these teams. Consider how the team will be recognized and how learning will be shared throughout the organization.

Redeployment of Resources

Normally, when an improvement team fulfills its project charter, the system undergoes some changes. These changes may cause displacement of people, redesign of work processes, or the need to train people with new or redesigned jobs.

Leaders should be as aware of the social and economic changes as they are of the technical changes. This is critical if the change is to be accepted and acted upon. As the teams perform their work, some principles of work design and redesign should be considered:

1. People should not be expected to "improve" themselves out of work. Leaders must take care of the social and economic consequences of job displacement. If people lose their jobs because of improvement, there will be increased resistance to change. A policy of attrition often is adopted to solve the expected short-term displacements. Sometimes the change is not acceptable to the person doing the job. This leads to the second principle.

2. People should be given choices. Leaders should be aware of the impact of displacement and should be prepared to explore alternatives for people affected by the change.

3. People who are displaced by a technical or economic change should be given some influence over their futures. Leaders should be careful to not take unilateral action in determining the future of displaced people.

EXERCISE 11.24

RESOURCE ALLOCATION

Discuss these issues as a leadership team. What are your views relative to these challenges when redeploying resources?

Removing Barriers and Obstacles

Many improvement efforts encounter obstacles as a team or individual attempts to accomplish the charter. These barriers and obstacles appear as technical problems, bureaucracy, regulations (both real and imagined), and people. Technical problems are the easiest obstacles to address. The other obstacles create frustration for individuals and teams. Why are we having this difficulty? We are just trying to improve our company! Why are these barriers in our way?

Change becomes a challenge when it cannot be controlled by someone who is affected by it. The natural defense is resistance. It has been noted that for every technical change in a process, there are social and economic changes as well. There are three phases of change:

1. Awareness (key role of the sponsor report leaders)
2. Acceptance
3. Action

Team leaders, sponsors, and others trying to remove obstacles from a change effort should understand this evolution of change. The awareness phase is critical to those bringing about change in an organization. In this phase, the people sponsoring and making the changes have the opportunity to educate those involved about the need for change and the expected results. A well-communicated explanation of *reasons to follow* will usually eliminate obstacles. If not, people need additional information and explanation.

Acceptance is voluntary. But it depends on having enough information to make a decision. Once there is acceptance, action follows naturally. When first encountering resistance to change, the sponsor or team leader should take care to provide the information that will equip people to make informed decisions.

If the resistance continues in the face of the facts, then the sponsor, or a higher-level manager, must deal with the resistance by participating in team discussions to learn about the sources of resistance.

Typical obstacles and barriers that can be expected by teams or individuals attempting improvement include

- Lack of time (real or perceived) to work on the change effort; critical in health care
- Lack of resources (meeting places, technical support, supplies, and so on)
- Problems with team dynamics
- Team members' fear of taking action
- Lack of subject matter knowledge in the team
- Management systems that impede change in the organization
- Cultural norms in the organization challenged by change (such as turf issues)
- Conflicts between multiple improvement efforts affecting the same area
- Disconnects due to language or poor communication
- Inability to take a systems view of the organization

Some ways that leaders can become aware of and deal with obstacles and barriers are

1. Provide sponsors from a higher level in the organization and make it clear that the sponsor is responsible for the success or failure of the improvement effort
2. Review biweekly sponsor reports from teams and offer guidance on progress (using the Model for Improvement as a road map)
3. Become more active and visible advocates for the change effort
4. Meet with the entire team periodically (four to six weeks) to better understand the barriers that have developed

Outline for an Agenda for a Sponsor/Team Review Meeting

- Review the project charter
- General review of the history of the team (sponsor reports)
- Detailed review of recent activities focusing around the cycles completed
- Discussion of barriers/group dynamics in the team
- Provide guidance as appropriate
- Discuss next steps for the team

EXERCISE 11.25

CONDUCT IMPROVEMENT TEAM REVIEW MEETING

Use the outline for an agenda for a sponsor/team review meeting to test with reviewing your improvement teams. (This exercise can be combined with 11.23.)

As teams and individuals are completing the work on their charters, the leadership team must keep in mind why the improvement efforts were initiated in the first place:

- To improve individual patient care and experience
- To learn from individual patients to improve population health
- To reduce per capita patient cost

As improvement efforts are completed, the leadership team should figure out how the results of the effort will affect the organization. Some issues to consider include

- What actions by leaders and managers are needed to reap the benefits of the improvement effort?
- What resources (budgets, positions, equipment and supplies, organization structures, and so forth) need to be modified due to the improvement effort?
- What permanent changes in the system need to be made to hold the gain? Examples include rewriting job descriptions, changing policies, updating procedure manuals, and reorganization of departments and staff.

If the leadership team does not effectively deal with these issues, the vision including gains from the improvement efforts will not be realized. Sometimes, resources made expendable from the improvement efforts should be invested in further improvements. For an organization increasing its market, these resources may be needed for running the business.

Chapter 9, "A Health Care Leader's Role in Building Knowledge," addressed the process of improving your ability to predict the results of change initiatives. As you improve this ability, you will be better able to design plans that are likely to be effective in achieving the results you seek. This process includes challenging your organization's underlying, and often unspoken, assumptions. By this method, you can create new normative theories that produce continuous learning and improvement. Leaders learn to reflect on experience, ask the right questions, and revise theories. Ackoff described four kinds of planning:

- *Reactive:* Planning is merely extrapolating from the past.
- *Inactive:* Day-to-day planning, what the British call "muddling through."
- *Preactive:* Proposes a road map drawn by experts who do not involve the people who must implement the plan.
- *Interactive:* Involves the whole organization and describes a systemic ideal future and then works out the steps to get from here to there. Ackoff called it backward planning. It makes use of all the tools presented in this book.

Keep in mind that this book aims to provide a set of tools to help you make your health care organization more effective and efficient to improve care while reducing costs. This leadership challenge is complex, made more difficult by payer policies that institute incentives for more care rather then better quality care. However, you have seen in these pages that leaders have been gaining results by practicing strategic intelligence and profound knowledge. We do not expect the ideas and practices described in this book to be applied all at once. They are tools to be mastered and applied time and again as you succeed in gaining the trust and collaboration of all those who will help you create a leaning organization that benefits patients, providers, and communities.

Table 11.9   Building a Learning Organization Component Evaluation

Components	Score = 0	Score = 2	Score = 4	Score = 6	Score = 8	Score = 10
Purpose and Practical Values	No written statements.	Statement exists.	Purpose and practical values defined and visible.	Communicated and understood by employees.	Used to align and guide the business. Roles of people are aligned.	Fully integrated into the structure.
Processes: Systems View	Work as a process is not understood.	Major processes and products have been documented.	Relationship between processes are documented.	Systems thinking is common.	Systems diagrams are used in business. People's roles are linked to the system.	Management systems have integrated the systems view.
Partnering	No formal partners.	Commodity supplier, based on specs and RFQ.	Preferred suppliers. Recognized quality traditional contractual relationship.	Value-added supplier. Distinctive competency. Traditional contractual relationship.	Alliance partnerships with suppliers. Joint projects. Sharing of knowledge. Relationship at start of project.	Strategic partnerships. Common vision. Mutual success.
People	People are viewed as necessary but replaceable in the bureaucratic organization.	People are appreciated for skills they bring. Training is viewed as an optional expense.	Knowledge and skills of people are important to the organization today. Training and education are necessary.	People are viewed as important to the purpose of the system. Development is important.	People have a defined role that allows them to contribute to the larger system purpose. People take responsibility for their development.	People understand how their role serves the larger purpose and their importance to the future of the organization and achieving the vision.

Results: System Measures	Financial data is viewed periodically.	Financial and other operational measures are used.	Family of measures is assembled aligned with purpose.	Measures are tracked over time. Leading indicators are used for prediction of future results.	Variation is understood; measures are aligned with individual roles.	Measures are integrated into management systems, values, and roles.
Information Sources: Aid to Foresight	Information is gathered on ad hoc, reactive basis.	System is based on passive information.	System is well documented and includes active sources.	Information is documented and communicated; industry leading sources are identified.	Comprehensive system with analysis/synthesis for decision making is used in planning and communication.	Information sources are synthesized to enable foresight and input to vision.
Visioning: Idealized Design of the Future	No vision.	Vision statement about being best in class.	Vision describes ideal results.	Vision is communicated and inspires stakeholders.	Vision guides behavior, strategy, developing, testing, and implementation of changes.	Idealized vision is realized; a new idealized design is created.

(continued)

Table 11.9   Continued

Components	Score = 0	Score = 2	Score = 4	Score = 6	Score = 8	Score = 10
Planning to Achieve the Purpose and Implement the Vision	No formal planning; reactive planning culture.	Planning for improvement is done on an informal basis; inactive.	A formal, documented process exists for proactive planning.	Integrated process identifies objectives, efforts, and resources.	All other planning processes are defined and linked within the organization and with partners.	Interactive backwards planning of ideal future system.
Leading and Integrating Change	No formal method exists to manage improvements.	Improvements are recognized as needed and resources assigned.	Learning and improvement utilizes charters and PDSAs routinely.	A formal method exists with leaders providing formal guidance for individuals and teams. Results are tracked overtime.	The impact of improvements are understood for the system and fits practical values. Improvement is linked to planning and other key business activities.	Improvement system is integrated in organization and regularly improved. Improvement is completely integrated into all aspects of operating and developing the business.
Motivating and Aligning People	Employees measured on following commands.	Use of financial incentives.	Supportive management and recognition.	Employees aligned with clear objectives.	Managers use all Five Rs to motivate.	The Five Rs are aligned with employee skills and values.

EXERCISE 11.26
LEARNING ORGANIZATION EVALUATION

Evaluate your progress toward creating a learning organization, check your progress on the evaluation grid.

SUMMARY

- It is important for you to understand your leadership philosophy and communicate it to others.
- Developing a statement of purpose and practical values that is congruent with your philosophy gives credibility to your actions in pursuit of the idealized vision for the future of the organization.
- Using the gap survey with people in the organization can help identify areas in which the leadership team can work to better model the practical values of the organization.
- The Strategic Intelligence Inventory should be taken by each member of the leadership team, the results displayed graphically and then discussed to ensure that the team is using strategic intelligence to guide the organization to the idealized vision.
- The Four Ps—purpose, practical values, people, and processes— should be used as a guide to define the vision of an idealized future for the organization.
- Driver diagrams can be utilized to effectively translate the vision into actionable charters to design and redesign the organization to move the organization to the idealized vision of the future.
- A charter approval form can be used to define the actionable charter using the first two questions from the Model for Improvement:
  a. What are we trying to accomplish?
  b. How will we know that a change is an improvement?

The individual or team that is given the charter can now answer the third question; what changes need to be made in order to make an improvement? The charter aligns and gives people the authority to effect change. People then *empower* themselves to develop, test, and implement changes.

- Managing individual and team projects is a key responsibility of the leadership team, acting to ensure that change efforts are properly resourced and barriers to execution mitigated or removed. The sponsor's job is to be the communication link between the leadership team and the people acting on the approved charters.
- The evaluation grid for strategic intelligence (SI) can provide feedback to the leadership team on how well they are deploying SI and the Four Ps. Gaps can be identified and plans made to more effectively utilize these ideas in the organization.

KEY TERMS

Driver diagram

Ideal future

Sponsor report

ENDNOTES

1. The X bar chart plots the averages of subgroup samples of data while the S chart plots the standard deviation of the sample subgroups. See Chapter 7 for a discussion of common cause and special cause variation and the patterns that define when special causes are present (see Figure 7.2).
2. To explore the thinking underlying the types, see Michael Maccoby, *Narcissistic Leaders, Who Succeeds and Who Fails* (Harvard Business School Press, 2007) and *The Leaders We Need, And What Makes Us Follow* (Harvard Business School Press, 2007).

Appendix

To discover what type or combination of types you are, take and score the Leadership Personality Survey, first published in *Narcissistic Leaders* by Michael Maccoby. Circle the number that represents your answer to each question:

Leadership Personality Survey

Table A.1 Leadership Personality Survey

How Well Does This Describe You?	Never	Almost Never	Seldom	Sometimes	Frequently	Almost Always
1 I want my work to further my own development.	0	1	3	6	10	15
2 I try to develop a vision for the ideal future of the institution.	0	1	3	6	10	15
3 I am an idealistic person.	0	1	3	6	10	15
4 I am satisfied at work if my job allows a great deal of autonomy.	0	1	3	6	10	15
5 I follow the rule that practice makes excellence.	0	1	3	6	10	15
6 I adapt easily to people I like.	0	1	3	6	10	15

(*continued*)

Table A.1 Continued

How Well Does This Describe You?	Never	Almost Never	Seldom	Sometimes	Frequently	Almost Always
7 I've developed my own view about what is right and wrong.	0	1	3	6	10	15
8 I see myself as a free agent.	0	1	3	6	10	15
9 I make my bosses into colleagues.	0	1	3	6	10	15
10 I adapt myself to continual change.	0	1	3	6	10	15
11 I feel I should take the initiative more.	0	1	3	6	10	15
12 Whatever my job, I try to provide high-quality work.	0	1	3	6	10	15
13 I try to keep my skills marketable.	0	1	3	6	10	15
14 I have a lot of aggressive energy I need to direct.	0	1	3	6	10	15
15 I keep my views to myself because I want to avoid an argument.	0	1	3	6	10	15
16 I put so much energy into responding to others that I feel I lose my sense of self.	0	1	3	6	10	15
17 The best boss for me is a good facilitator.	0	1	3	6	10	15
18 I try to be tough so I won't seem too soft.	0	1	3	6	10	15
19 I am bothered when there is a lack of neatness.	0	1	3	6	10	15
20 I find that the market gives me feedback on my value.	0	1	3	6	10	15

Table A.1 Continued

How Well Does This Describe You?	Never	Almost Never	Seldom	Sometimes	Frequently	Almost Always
21 I have conversations with myself to clarify what I should do.	0	1	3	6	10	15
22 The best boss for me is like a good father who recognizes my achievements.	0	1	3	6	10	15
23 I want to feel appreciated.	0	1	3	6	10	15
24 I try to keep my options open.	0	1	3	6	10	15
25 I compare myself to highly successful people.	0	1	3	6	10	15
26 I like to collect things.	0	1	3	6	10	15
27 I believe the best decision will result from consensus.	0	1	3	6	10	15
28 I would rather be loved than admired.	0	1	3	6	10	15
29 I like to feel needed by people I care about.	0	1	3	6	10	15
30 What I like about games is the challenge to improve my personal score.	0	1	3	6	10	15
31 I admire creative geniuses.	0	1	3	6	10	15
32 I have difficulty completing projects on time because I want my work to be perfect.	0	1	3	6	10	15
33 Loyalty does not get in my way of doing what is best to succeed.	0	1	3	6	10	15
34 I feel alone and isolated.	0	1	3	6	10	15
35 I am thorough rather than quick.	0	1	3	6	10	15

(continued)

Table A.1 Continued

How Well Does This Describe You?	Never	Almost Never	Seldom	Sometimes	Frequently	Almost Always
36 I don't give in when I feel I am in the right.	0	1	3	6	10	15
37 I trust people.	0	1	3	6	10	15
38 I use organizations as instruments to achieve my goals.	0	1	3	6	10	15
39 I keep up with the latest trends.	0	1	3	6	10	15
40 I follow my ideas despite what people say.	0	1	3	6	10	15
41 My sense of security comes from supportive family and friends.	0	1	3	6	10	15
42 I judge people according to strict moral standards.	0	1	3	6	10	15
43 Before I accept an idea, I check it out with people I respect.	0	1	3	6	10	15
44 The best boss for me makes the workgroup into a kind of family.	0	1	3	6	10	15
45 I feel I get taken in by people I've trusted.	0	1	3	6	10	15
46 I like to help people.	0	1	3	6	10	15
47 I define quality in terms of what experts value.	0	1	3	6	10	15
48 I don't act until I have fully weighed the alternatives.	0	1	3	6	10	15
49 I evaluate behavior in terms of what is considered appropriate by the people I respect.	0	1	3	6	10	15
50 I create meaning for myself and others at work.	0	1	3	6	10	15

Table A.1   Continued

How Well Does This Describe You?	Never	Almost Never	Seldom	Sometimes	Frequently	Almost Always
51 I am building a network of others who share my values.	0	1	3	6	10	15
52 I enjoy loving more than being loved.	0	1	3	6	10	15
53 I enjoy being part of a cooperative group.	0	1	3	6	10	15
54 I feel better when I save rather than spend.	0	1	3	6	10	15
55 I would rather be admired than liked.	0	1	3	6	10	15
56 I am very tolerant about what others do.	0	1	3	6	10	15
57 I like bringing people together.	0	1	3	6	10	15
58 I sense when people are working against me.	0	1	3	6	10	15
59 I spend a lot of time on details.	0	1	3	6	10	15
60 I like to associate with the top people.	0	1	3	6	10	15
61 I spend a lot of time chatting with my friends.	0	1	3	6	10	15
62 My creativity depends on maintaining my freedom.	0	1	3	6	10	15
63 I enjoy interactions where I can learn something new.	0	1	3	6	10	15
64 I feel I give in too much.	0	1	3	6	10	15
65 Once I start talking I tend to go on.	0	1	3	6	10	15
66 I approach my work as a means to a self-fulfilling life.	0	1	3	6	10	15

(continued)

Table A.1 Continued

How Well Does This Describe You?	Never	Almost Never	Seldom	Sometimes	Frequently	Almost Always
67 I try to know everything about everything that has an impact on my institution.	0	1	3	6	10	15
68 I like to have a schedule and keep to it.	0	1	3	6	10	15
69 The best thing about playing games is having a good time with my friends.	0	1	3	6	10	15
70 I seek out people who can contribute to my plans.	0	1	3	6	10	15
71 I test out my ideas systematically.	0	1	3	6	10	15
72 To be successful, I try to look good.	0	1	3	6	10	15
73 People at work are either with me or against me.	0	1	3	6	10	15
74 I like to keep up with old friends.	0	1	3	6	10	15
75 I rely on certain people who care about me.	0	1	3	6	10	15
76 I put my own spirit into my products and creations.	0	1	3	6	10	15
77 My sense of security is based on my reputation in my field.	0	1	3	6	10	15
78 My self-esteem depends on being seen as successful.	0	1	3	6	10	15
79 I like to develop ways to improve efficiency.	0	1	3	6	10	15
80 I admire people who have helped those in need.	0	1	3	6	10	15

Following is a key to scoring the leadership personality questionnaire. Write your answer (numerical score) to each question in Table A.2.

Table A.2   Scoring Chart for Personality Survey

1	___	2	___	3	___	4	___
8	___	7	___	6	___	5	___
10	___	9	___	11	___	12	___
13	___	14	___	15	___	19	___
16	___	21	___	18	___	22	___
17	___	25	___	23	___	26	___
20	___	31	___	28	___	30	___
24	___	34	___	29	___	32	___
27	___	38	___	37	___	35	___
33	___	40	___	41	___	36	___
39	___	50	___	44	___	42	___
43	___	52	___	45	___	48	___
47	___	55	___	46	___	54	___
49	___	58	___	53	___	59	___
51	___	60	___	57	___	65	___
56	___	62	___	61	___	68	___
63	___	67	___	64	___	71	___
66	___	70	___	69	___	74	___
72	___	73	___	75	___	77	___
78	___	76	___	80	___	79	___

TOTAL:

___	___	___	___
Adaptive	Visionary	Caring	Exacting

To understand your personality type, turn to the section Understanding Leadership Personality.

Social Character Questionnaire

Your personality is also shaped by your social character. We are in a transition period where bureaucratic and interactive social characters coexist in the workplace. Which are you most like? You may have attitudes that clearly belong to one or the other or both types. Answer these questions to find out. How much do you agree with these statements?

Table A.3 Social Character Questionnaire

		Not at all	Very little	Some- what	Very much
1	It is important for me to have a clear role in my organization.	0	1	3	4
2	I'd like to work for an organization that values loyalty.	0	1	3	4
3	I can benefit from continual change.	0	1	3	4
4	I see myself as a free agent, alert to better opportunities.	0	1	3	4
5	I want to be part of a team of people who share the same values.	0	1	3	4
6	I work at continually developing myself intellectually, emotionally, and physically.	0	1	3	4
7	Leaders should be people with the most experience.	0	1	3	4
8	I care more that team members share a common purpose than that they have the same values.	0	1	3	4
9	I want to work in an organization that values seniority.	0	1	3	4
10	I am continually developing my network.	0	1	3	4
11	I want a job description with clear lines of authority.	0	1	3	4
12	I like to work in a team where leadership shifts to the person with the appropriate skills.	0	1	3	4
13	I like interacting with people throughout the world on the Internet.	0	1	3	4
14	I prefer to be on a team where the leader is a facilitator rather than a boss.	0	1	3	4

Table A.3   Continued

		Not at all	Very little	Some-what	Very much
15	I use the Internet regularly to find information about people.	0	1	3	4
16	My goal at work is to meet the expectations set for me.	0	1	3	4
17	I care more that the work we produce is excellent than that it satisfies a customer.	0	1	3	4
18	The best boss is like a good father or mother.	0	1	3	4
19	I can change my image to fit the situation.	0	1	3	4
20	My goal at work is to be respected as an expert.	0	1	3	4

Scoring of Social Character Questionnaire

Write your answer to each question in Table A.4.

Table A.4   Scoring for Social Character Questionnaire

1	_____	3	_____
2	_____	4	_____
5	_____	6	_____
7	_____	8	_____
9	_____	10	_____
11	_____	12	_____
16	_____	13	_____
17	_____	14	_____
18	_____	15	_____
20	_____	19	_____

TOTAL: **TOTAL:**

_____   _____

This is your   This is your
<u>Bureaucratic</u> Score   <u>Interactive</u> Score

Which social character best describes you?
Compare your score to that of those you lead or to members of your team.
What do the differences mean? Do they cause conflicts at work?

Understanding Leadership Personality

The personalities of leaders color their relationships and influence their strategic decisions and behaviors. Personality focuses the leader's attention on aspects of the future and may also narrow that focus. Personality shapes the types of visions that are meaningful to leaders and the way they think about organizational systems. Leaders' personalities direct them to the types of people they consider as partners in accomplishing their visions—and the way they recruit, motivate, and empower them.

The Maccoby Leadership Personality Survey provides insight into the way a leader's personality interacts with an organization and the larger society. It is a survey, meaning that it is wide ranging, offering a full consideration of the aspects of personality affecting leadership. Just as a survey of land has as one of its goals the creation of a map to make the landscape more understandable, the Maccoby Leadership Personality Survey generates a diagram to assist in making the leader's personality more understandable. Only when we understand our personalities are we able to improve them and to become more productive.

You can map your questionnaire scores on this diamond.

Figure A.1   Graph for Personality Type Questionnaire

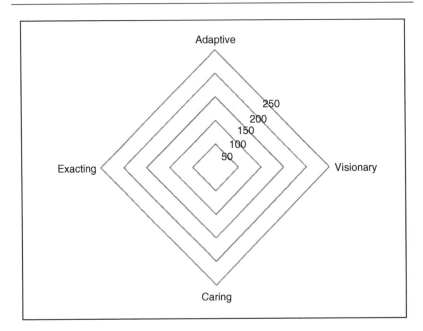

Your highest score is your dominant type, the next highest your secondary type. Keep in mind that each person is unique. However, the types are patterns of value-drives or motivational values that we often observe. You can use the results as a frame for understanding yourself and others.

The personality of every person—and therefore every leader—is a combination or blend of types that work together as a system. To understand these personality systems, the following pages present, first, the four types and then considers them in their various combinations with the other types—with an emphasis on leadership.

For some people, a single type is clearly dominant but never to the total exclusion of factors related to the other types. For other people, one type may be dominant and blended with a clear secondary type. Many combinations of the four types are possible.

The Four Primary Leadership Personality Types

1. Caring
2. Visionary
3. Exacting
4. Adaptive

The Caring (Freud's Erotic) Leadership Personality

Figure A.2   Caring Personality

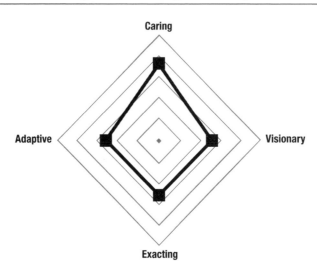

The most important value is loving and being loved. Leaders of this type want to help and care for people. They also want to be seen by others as helpers, to be recognized for their good deeds and to be loved and appreciated, more than respected or admired. They want to believe in other people and to have the trust they naturally place in others be rewarded by reciprocal trust and personal loyalty.

The caring type dominates the social services; the caring fields—teaching, nursing, social work, mental health, and therapy—and service industries; careers that involve personal management, nurturing creativity and growth, and encouraging others to make more of their lives. They keep our social services running on both an organizational and personal level by teaching our children; caring for the elderly; helping displaced, homeless, or poor people; and on a smaller scale, setting up this friend with that one, lending a hand with moving, or coming over to cook dinner for a sick colleague. They are drawn to organizations that pursue social causes or have social consciences.

Caring types are typically good listeners and are receptive to others and open to hearing about their experiences, ideas, and emotions. They like to share news of personal events and quite naturally expect others to want to do the same.

They never like to say no to a favor. They thrive on service and cooperation and trust and rely on friends and family for a sense of security. When caring types rise to leadership positions, it's usually in the caring fields, rather than innovative or high-tech companies. However, they can be found in military leadership where they mentor and forge strong bonds of friendship. They also shine as musicians and performers who stimulate love in their audiences. They can also be found in technical roles as helpers to other leaders.

Table A.5   Strengths and Weaknesses, Caring Personality

Strengths	Weaknesses
Caring	Dependency
Bringing people together	Gullibility and disillusionment
Reinforcing social interdependence	Inability to make tough decisions
Service and cooperation	Fear of taking a stand
Trust	Excesses of emotion
Stimulating love	The need for everyone to like them
Devoted	Submissive
Optimistic	Wishful thinking
Sensitive	Easily perceive rejection
Helpful	Smothering or intrusive

The Visionary (Freud's Narcissistic) Leadership Personality

Figure A.3   Visionary Personality

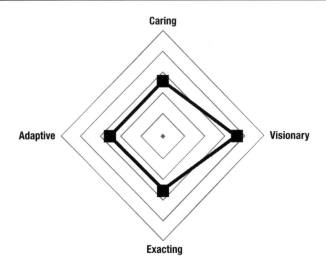

The productive leaders of this type impress us as personalities who disrupt the status quo and bring about change.

Visionaries have very little or no psychic demands that they have to do the right thing. Freed from these internal constraints, they are forced to answer for themselves what is right, to decide what they value and what, in effect, gives them a sense of meaning. The productive ones create their own vision, with a sense of purpose that not only engages them but may also inspire others to follow them. This vision may be either ethical or unethical, for the common good or for personal power. The visions of unproductive narcissists may be grandiose or irrational, isolating them from others.

Visionaries are accustomed to listening to themselves, their inner voices. They may debate different sides of an issue (for example, "to be or not to be"), finally reaching a decision about what to do and the best way to do it. They tend to block out the voices of others.

Without the support of others, it's easy to see how visionaries have a highly developed "me against the world" way of looking at things. It often comes out as paranoia, a heightened awareness of danger, which may be realistic, given narcissistic ambition, competitiveness, and unbridled, aggressive energy. There's not a lot of gray area in the visionary-narcissistic view of the world. You are either a friend or a foe, for or against the vision, which has become merged with the narcissist's sense of self.

Because they have not internalized a strong superego in childhood, they are able to be more aggressive than other types.

Productive visionaries are not limited to any particular field; you can find them in almost any field and in any domain. They may not change the entire world (though some certainly have), but they may reinvent their part of the world.

Table A.6 Strengths and Weaknesses, Visionary Personality

Strengths	Weaknesses
Visioning to change the world and create meaning that others can share	Extreme sensitivity to criticism
Independent thinking/risk taking	Not listening
Passion about ideas	Paranoia
Charisma	Extreme competitiveness
Voracious learning	Anger and put-downs
Perseverance	Exaggeration
Alertness to threats	Lack of self-knowledge
Sense of humor	Isolation
	Grandiosity

The Exacting (Freud's Obsessive) Leadership Personality

Figure A.4   Exacting Personality

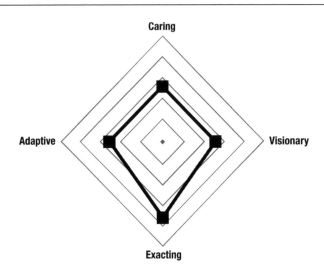

Exacting leadership personalities are inner-directed. They live by the rules, and the rules are usually determined by internalized, parental figures, forging a strict conscience or following "the way things have always been done around here." People of this type are motivated to live up to the high standards and ideals they set for themselves and to show, at all times, that they fit the ideal of "good child" to internalized parental figures. When they fail or rebel against these internalized demands, they feel guilty.

They are the conservatives who preserve order and maintain moral values with a strong work ethic. They focus on the importance of right and wrong, whether at work or in their friendships. Once they believe in someone or something, they stick to it, showing loyalty. They want good, orderly fashion in everything they touch or do, whether it's in their well-kept closets or work spaces or in how they organize their time. The most productive of these types are systematic. They systematically break a task down into its components and set out to tackle it, one bit at a time.

They are the kinds of people who say, "If you're going to do anything, you should do it right." Exacting experts see work as performance, a way to meet a standard and not necessarily be helpful to anyone. In the past, they were the independent farmers and craftsmen. Today, they are doctors, engineers, financial experts, accountants, scientists, researchers, technicians, and craftsmen, like electricians, bricklayers, and carpenters. They are also the majority of middle managers and some top managers, especially CFOs, COOs, and some CEOs.

An exacting type may make it to the top of a corporation and take on a leadership role, but they are most effective in a company that is itself exacting, such as a company in manufacturing or retail that is conservative and focused on the bottom line, whose success depends on creating processes that improve quality and cut costs. They can also be effective in a government agency.

Table A.7   Strengths and Weaknesses, Exacting Personality

Strengths	Weaknesses
Systematic	Resists anything new or different
Maintain order and stability	Gets mired in details and rules, loses sight of overall goals
Preserve tradition	
Loyal and faithful to their commitments	More concerned with doing things in the right way than doing the right thing
Exacting standards, high-quality work	
Disciplined and diligent	Control freaks, paper-pushing, bean-counting bureaucrats
Determined	
Responsible and accountable	Judgmental, stubborn, stingy, and extremely neat and clean
	Always right, know-it-alls

The Adaptive (Fromm's Marketing) Leadership Personality

Figure A.5   Adaptive Personality

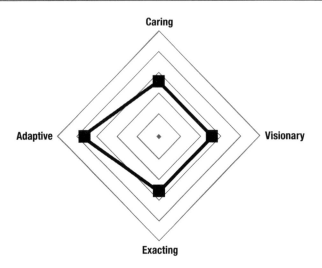

These leaders operate by radar, sensing what the market wants and needs and then either developing themselves to fit it or just conforming to it. Their self-esteem or self-valuation comes from what could be called a personal stock that goes up and down depending on what they're selling, including their accomplishments, how well they align themselves with key people, a client or account base, good looks and style, new skills and expertise, or "whatever," as they are fond of saying. Everything they do is relative; it needs to meet the approval of other people. They rarely use the words "right" or "wrong" (as does the exacting type); they want their behavior to be "appropriate." They intuitively know how to adapt to changes in the marketplace and are not as unsettled by upheaval in the corporate or economic climate as others are. They see change as an opportunity for success and fun.

The most productive adaptive personalities are interactive self-developers. They think of their life and career as continuing education, a chance to pick up new skills. They continually learn and grow, intellectually and emotionally. They are the types who want to do well and feel and look good. They exercise, diet, talk to therapists, organize reading and study groups and take classes. They are some of the most productive freelancers, setting their own goals and working well on their own; they are a big part of the current trend toward self-employment and are excellent at self-promotion. However, they also are natural networkers and team players and enjoy interacting with people like themselves.

This type does well in all manner of sales professions: real estate, public relations, advertising, publicity, events planning, venture capital, and money-raising. They are effective in consulting, technical design, acting, the arts, publishing, and entertainment. They increasingly play a part in the legal and medical professions because of their ability to bring people together. They are often chosen as school principals and college or university presidents, because they make all the different interest groups feel understood and supported. They build coalitions that don't insult anyone. They are the most effective facilitators, and the best such leaders partner with innovative visionaries and exacting operational leaders.

Table A.8   Strengths and Weaknesses, Adaptive Personality

Strengths	Weaknesses
Intuitively adapting to changes in the marketplace	Indecisive, noncommittal
Superior networking skills	No center, no inner core that directs them
Continual reinvention	No lasting commitments to their work or to people
Self-marketing	
Interactive	Anxiety and uncertainty hang over them, the nagging question "Is this the appropriate answer? Am I doing OK? Is this working?"
Natural mediators and interpreters between other personalities	
Tolerant	Indifferent
Adaptable	

Leadership Personality Examples

Every person is a blend of personality types. Many people listed in this table have strong characteristics of types in addition to the column in which they are listed. Individual types were determined primarily by study of biographies, these people's writings, observations by peers, and observations by authors.

Table A.9   Leadership Personality Examples

	Caring	Visionary	Exacting	Adaptive
Past Business Leaders	Darwin Smith of Kimberly-Clark, David Maxwell of Fannie Mae, Kris McDivitt of Patagonia	John D. Rockefeller, Henry Ford, Andrew Carnegie, Walt Disney, Jack Welch, Helena Rubinstein, Mary Kay	Bill Hewlett, Sam Walton	Carly Fiorina
Present Business Leaders	Howard Schultz of Starbucks	Bill Gates, Larry Ellison, Steve Jobs, Martha Stewart, Oprah Winfrey	Michael Dell, Mark Hurd	John Chambers, Bob Iger, Jeff Immelt, Richard Parsons
Arts	Vincent van Gogh, Norman Rockwell	Frank Lloyd Wright, Frank Gehry, Leonardo da Vinci, Michelangelo, Pablo Picasso	Ansel Adams, Georges Seurat	Andy Warhol, Henri de Toulouse-Lautrec
Thought Leaders	Elias Porter, Thomas Gordon	Ayn Rand, Sigmund Freud, Albert Einstein	Alfred Nobel, Carl Rogers, John Muir, Louis Pasteur, Jonas Salk	Paul Hersey, Malcolm Gladwell
U.S. Presidents	Jimmy Carter, Ulysses S. Grant	Abraham Lincoln, FDR, Richard Nixon, Ronald Reagan, Bill Clinton, Barack Obama	George H. W. Bush, Woodrow Wilson	John F. Kennedy, George W. Bush

Table A.9 Continued

	Caring	Visionary	Exacting	Adaptive
Political Leaders	Gandhi, Mother Teresa, Nelson Mandela	Napoleon, Churchill, de Gaulle, Fidel Castro, Nicolas Sarkozy	Al Gore, John McCain, Gordon Brown, Vladimir Putin	Tony Blair, David Cameron, Sarah Palin
U.S. Military Leaders	Ulysses S. Grant, Norman Schwarzkopf	Douglas MacArthur, George Patton	George Washington, Dwight Eisenhower	David Petraeus, Colin Powell

Combinations of Types

Characteristics of the four personality types are, to some degree, present in every person. Neither the visionary nor the adaptive internalize parental commands about right and wrong. But while adaptives identify with peers and seek consensus about moral decisions, visionaries determine their own sense of what is right and wrong. A focus on the four types is a useful starting point, but a consideration of the various combinations of types reveals subtleties and the ways the types work together as a system to form unique personalities.

Table A.10 Summary of Productive Mixed Leadership Types

		Dominant Type			
		Caring	**Visionary**	**Exacting**	**Adaptive**
Secondary Type	Caring	Caring	Institution Builder	Exacting Teacher	Consensus Builder
	Visionary	Humanitarian	Visionary	Process Creator	Guru
	Exacting	Counselor	Strategic Leader	Exacting	Technical Salesperson
	Adaptive	Helper	Entrepreneur	Technical Consultant	Adaptive

CARING-Dominant Mixed Leadership Types

CARING-Visionary (Humanitarian)

This type is a humanitarian leader, attuned to the needs of others and ready to take up a social cause or effort for the betterment of others who are in need. They will pour enormous effort into even long-shot chances to help the disadvantaged, often soliciting the help of others in their efforts. Some, like Mother Teresa, begin by caring for individuals in need and then create an order and mission to continue the work.

The unproductive type can let the needs of others drive their business or financial decisions and may give to others to the point that they lose their capacity to give more.

Figure A.6   Caring-Visionary Personality

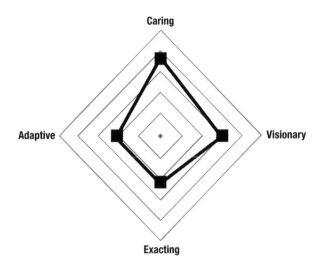

CARING-Exacting (Counselor)

Figure A.7   Caring-Exacting Personality

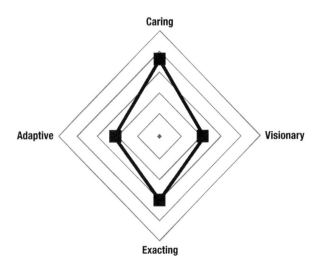

The productive leader is the caring but exacting mentor or good counselor, sensing the needs of others, offering advice, and helping other people to make their own decisions. This is also the prototype of the good mother, caring, hardworking, and concerned with the health of her children. This combination can make effective general practitioner doctors and nurses. Some, with strategic intelligence, have done well as military commanders, like Ulysses S. Grant and Dwight D. Eisenhower. Caring artists like Wynton Marsalis bring out the best in their collaborators.

The unproductive version is a type that worries obsessively about health issues or about whether they are loved. This type can be too easily manipulated because they fear losing love and can be too trusting.

CARING-Adaptive (Helper)

Figure A.8   Caring-Adaptive Personality

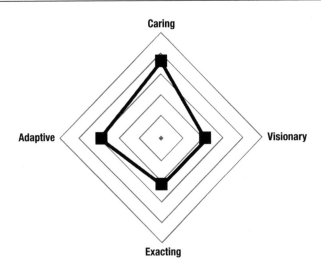

The productive leader is a helper, sensitive and receptive to the needs of many others at one time or the collective needs of a small group. They excel in situations where they can support a small group of people or a team. Many psychotherapists are this type.

The unproductive types are constantly looking for a fulfilling relationship. They have many infatuations where they believe they have found themselves, but they inevitably decide they have lost themselves.

VISIONARY-Dominant Mixed Leadership Types

VISIONARY-Caring (Institution Builder)

Figure A.9   Visionary-Caring Personality

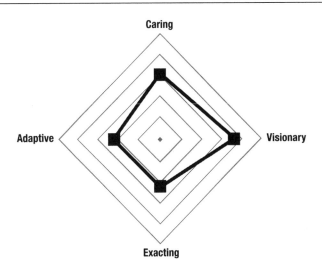

The productive version is the institution builder, who not only builds an institution, like a hospital or school, but leads it and cares for the people, like Father William Wasson who created Nuestros Pequeños Hermanos, an orphanage in nine countries. Some are creative musicians or actors like Orson Welles or Marlon Brando. There are also organizational leaders of this type who need to partner with exacting types, because they ignore processes and details, focusing on caring for the people who sign on to their vision.

The unproductive version is the Don Juan or Mata Hari type, seductive and exploitative, using sensitivity to others' needs to find paths open to manipulation and gaining personal power.

VISIONARY-Exacting (Strategic Leader)

The productive version is what Freud considered the best strategic leader, combining vision and systematic approaches to implementation. They want results to be accomplished according to a plan and see the planning process as rehearsal and preparation for action. Jack Welch is a good example of this type. Freud also thought himself this type. Others are Larry Ellison and Bill Gates.

Figure A.10   Visionary-Exacting Personality

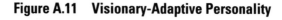

The unproductive version is the authoritarian bureaucrat, paranoid, hoarding, and without a creative vision. They lack interpersonal sensitivity. Rather, their vision is total control and domination.

VISIONARY-Adaptive (Entrepreneur)

Figure A.11   Visionary-Adaptive Personality

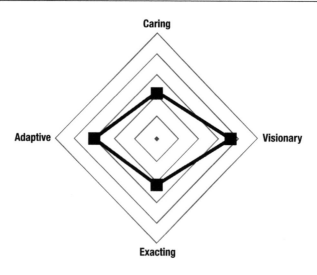

The productive version uses marketing traits in order to recruit others without being controlled by others or trying to please them. Their visions are adapted to people's needs. Jan Carlzon was this type of leader at Scandinavian Airlines in the 1980s and 1990s. Steve Jobs and Barack Obama are other examples. This is the emerging type of new entrepreneur.

The unproductive individuals tend to suffer from frustrated grandiosity, as they continually crank out visions that no one buys, trying to find new and better ways to convince people that their latest project or idea is different from past, failed attempts.

EXACTING-Dominant Mixed Leadership Types

EXACTING-Caring (Exacting Teacher)

Figure A.12   Exacting-Caring Personality

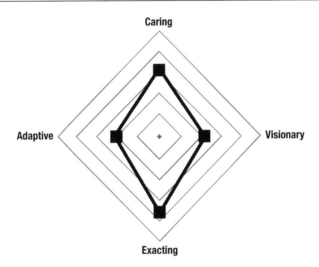

The productive leader is the exacting teacher and, in business, the person who can identify problems and recommend specific steps to remedy them. As a metaphor, they are ideal clinicians and careful doctors. This type is also attracted to professional roles that require people to be systematic and thorough but still want to help people succeed.

The unproductive version is the dependent but rigid type. As bureaucrats, they are servile to bosses but unbending to clients and subordinates.

EXACTING-Visionary (Process Creator)

Figure A.13   Exacting-Visionary Personality

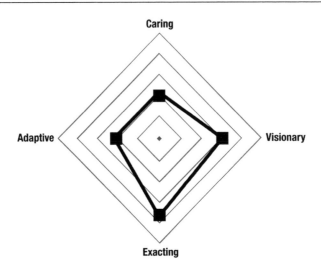

The productive version is the process creator, the leader who can create structure and order in systems that seem otherwise unmanageable. These types believe that making the organization run more efficiently is a great vision. It is likely that they are conscientiously attempting to improve the organization but not change the world.

The unproductive version becomes a controlling micromanager, insisting on compliance with processes and rules that do not contribute to meaningful outcomes.

EXACTING-Adaptive (Technical Consultant)

Productive leaders are technical consultants with an emphasis on what they have to offer, rather than what others need from them. They focus on developing their skills and looking good, adapting to the market in order to succeed. They are careful to walk the walk, talk the talk, and be informed on all the latest trends that may have an effect on their jobs or their customers.

The unproductive version is the proverbial "solution in search of a problem." They are so eager to apply their knowledge and expertise that every situation seems to fit in exactly with what they know.

Figure A.14 Exacting-Adaptive Personality

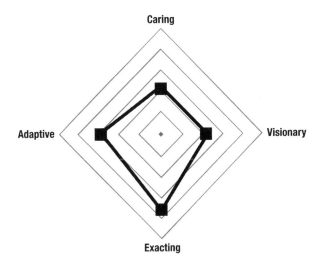

ADAPTIVE-Dominant Mixed Leadership Types

ADAPTIVE-Caring (Consensus Builder)

Figure A.15 Adaptive-Caring Personality

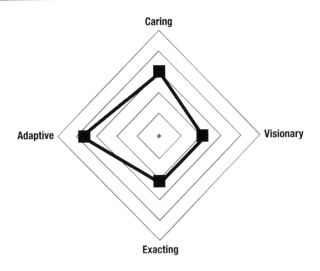

The productive leader is the consensus builder. Because they value the needs of many people at the same time, they naturally try to get people to see things from each others' viewpoints. They focus on finding and creating areas of agreement, while gaining some economic and social advantage from helping others. This type is particularly good at sales and public relations.

The unproductive types believe that if they look right and give others what they seem to want, they will be loved. They may run into trouble by agreeing with too many people and leaving the impression that they do not have an opinion or standard of their own. They are the perpetual consumers, who believe that they will find satisfaction through buying or experiencing what is fashionable.

ADAPTIVE-Visionary (Guru)

Figure A.16 Adaptive-Visionary Personality

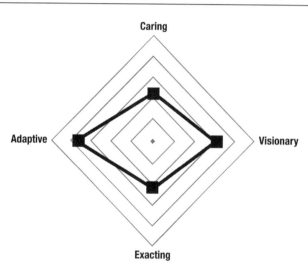

The productive leader is the guru who is quick to assess the situation and package a customized solution. Because they value both speed and novelty, they are often among the early adopters of new technology, but they can tire of it quickly. In marketing or public relations, they can be the extremely innovative ones, who create the perception of new needs in the market.

The unproductive types are unsure of their ideas, continually looking to others to affirm them. They may also suffer from multitasking, overcommitment to multiple visions or projects, or continually changing visions.

ADAPTIVE-Exacting (Technical Salesperson)

Figure A.17   Adaptive-Exacting Personality

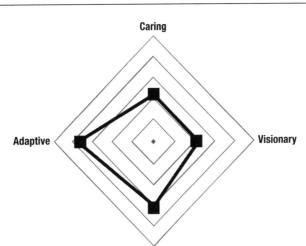

The productive type is especially effective as a technical salesperson or leader of a technical organization or team. Professionals of this type are able to build useful networks and provide value for their clients because they listen well to problems and are systematic in following through. They keep up on the latest information and make good use of it.

The unproductive types can be obsessive about getting more information than they can use. They compulsively surf the Internet or wade through the latest books, magazines, and newspapers in search of the "new."

Mixed Type and Social Character

Personality types are best understood in the context of social character. The socialization process and relationship to the dominant means of production in a society have a significant influence on the meaning that people create for themselves and their value-drives. For that reason, the same type will mean something different in each social character.

Farming-Craft Social Character

Figure A.18   Farming-Craft Social Character

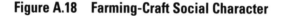

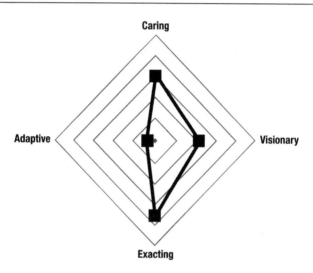

The prototype of the farming-craft social character is exacting-dominant with a secondary of caring. Fromm and Maccoby did not find any adaptive types in their study of Mexican villagers. The visionaries were the entrepreneurs who were changing the culture. The productive version of this type is the traditional self-sufficient local producer of agricultural or material goods. In the farming-craft social character, the dominant personality types tend to be expressed as follows:

Caring: Love is directed to family members or apprentices.

Visionary: Entrepreneurs start new businesses and invest in new technologies.

Exacting: In traditional work, done independently or, in the case of farming, with help from family members.

Bureaucratic Social Character

Figure A.19   Bureaucratic Social Character

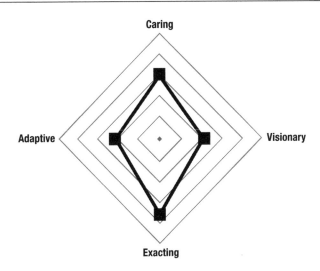

In the bureaucratic social character, the prototype personality is similar to farming-craft, but with a little more strength of the visionary and the emergence of the adaptive. This type is related to a means of production with strong organizational roles and rules. Production is typically either formatted, manual work, or more abstract office work, using words and symbols, rather than the hand tools of the farming-craft mode of production. In the bureaucratic social character, the dominant personality types tend to be expressed as follows:

Caring: A mentor or a helper to authorities. These caring types give loyalty to organizations or persons they feel are loyal to them.

Visionary: Introducing innovative or disruptive ideas within bureaucratic structures. Creation of new organizations to seize and control new markets.

Exacting: Creation and adherence to structure and process. Organization of workflows and systems in linear or hierarchical manners. Becoming an expert to gain status and power in the bureaucracy.

Adaptive: First to respond to the visionaries. Seeking networks for support.

Interactive Social Character

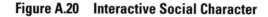

Figure A.20   Interactive Social Character

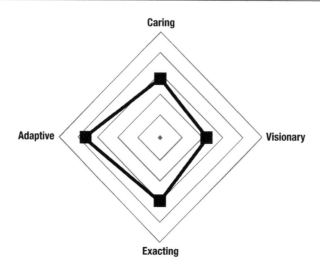

The prototype of the interactive social character is adaptive-dominant, followed by exacting, caring, and visionary. The moderately productive version of this type is the average personality in the knowledge-service age. They smoothly fit right into the team-based organization of modern knowledge-work.

In the interactive social character, the dominant personality types tend to be expressed as follows:

Caring: Focused on a person or group. Easily directed away to a new person or group that promises greater gain or enjoyment.

Visionary: The "change the world" mentality. Dissatisfaction with the status quo and a desire to recruit people to their change efforts.

Exacting: Solving problems or selling services. Creating holistic systems that adapt to business needs and make information available across functions.

Adaptive: Sensing shifts in market forces and trends, networking, forming and reforming groups to do project-based work. Seeking new ways to add value. Looking for ways to increase their own marketability.

Glossary

The purpose of this glossary is for our readers to share with the authors the meanings of the concepts in this book. Health care has a language of its own. In this glossary, we define how particular words have been used as terms in the book. Mortimer Adler has noted, "If the author uses a word in one meaning, and the reader reads it in another, words have passed between them, but they have not come to terms. Where there is unresolved ambiguity in communication, there is no communication, or at best communication must be incomplete."[1]

ADE

> An adverse drug event describes harm caused by the use of given medications. According to the Agency for Healthcare Research and Quality of the U.S. Department of Health and Human Services, over 770,000 people are injured or die each year in hospitals from adverse drug events (ADEs). These ADEs may cost up to $5.6 million each year per hospital depending on hospital size. This estimate does not include ADEs causing admissions, malpractice and litigation costs, or the costs of injuries to patients.

Albumin (Alb)

> Albumin is the main protein of plasma; it binds water, cations (such as Ca^{2+}, Na^+, and K^+), fatty acids, hormones, bilirubin, thyroxine (T4), and drugs (including barbiturates)—its main function is to regulate the colloidal osmotic pressure of blood.

Alignment

Alignment is the design of elements of a system so that together they optimally contribute to achieving the purpose and vision of the system. These elements may be values, strategic objectives, improvement efforts, programs, processes, roles, responsibilities, or people.

Attribution Theory

Describes the tendency for observers to underestimate situational (system) influences and overestimate motives and personality (individual) traits as the cause of behavior.

Big Five, The

Psychological research indicates there are five temperamental traits that appear to be genetically determined, but at least to some degree can be strengthened. The Big Five are openness; agreeableness; emotional stability; conscientiousness; extraversion versus introversion.

Bottleneck

Key leverage points that are constraints in the work system of an organization.

Building the Foundation of the Learning Organization, aka Quality as a Business Strategy (QBS)

These methods include purpose, the organization viewed as a system, measures of the systems, system to obtain information (focused on customers), planning, and managing individual and team improvement efforts.

Bureaucratic Social Character

The social character of people whose attitudes and values motivate them to adapt to industrial bureaucracies. They tend to be inner-directed, precise, methodical, and obsessive, and they identify with parental authority; versus the interactive social character.

Chain Reaction

The Deming quality concept that an improvement in quality leads to decreases in costs due to less rework, fewer mistakes, fewer delays and snags, and a better use of time and materials. These improvements lead to improved productivity, that leads to capturing the market with better products and services and lower prices for the consumer.

Collaboration

Collaboration means working with others, in spite of differences, to achieve a common goal. In a complex organization with differing types of authority, knowledge, and work, collaboration is essential to address challenges and threats that cannot be solved by one profession or part of the organization.

Common Cause(s) of Variation

Those causes that are inherent in the process over time, affect everyone working in the process, and affect all outcomes of the process.

Consensus

Decision making when everyone's ideas are explored through dialogue; team members understand the views of other team members to the extent that all can support the decision of the group. This process engages all team members and generates support by all members to implement the decision.

Constraint

Anything that restricts the throughput of a system. A constraint within an organization can be any resource where the demand for that resource is greater than its available capacity. In order to increase the throughput in a system, the constraints should be identified, exploited if possible, and removed if necessary.

Control Chart

A statistical tool used to distinguish between variation in a process due to common causes and variation due to special causes.

It is constructed by obtaining measurements of some characteristic of a process and grouping the data by time period, location,
or other variables that describe the process.

Control Limits

Control limits are usually horizontal lines drawn on a control
chart, typically at a distance of ± 3 standard deviations of the
plotted statistic from the statistic's mean. Control limits should
not be confused with tolerance limits or specifications, which
are completely independent of the distribution of the plotted
sample statistic.

County Council (Sweden)

A county council, or *landsting,* is an elected assembly of a
county in Sweden. It is a political entity, elected by the county
electorate, and has responsibilities for the public health care
system in that county.

Craft Mode of Production

The craft mode of production describes a way of organizing
work and relationships based on the use of hand tools to produce objects and services. Master craftsmen train apprentices.
The craft mode arose prior to the introduction of industrial
production, the assembly line, and bureaucratic organization,
whose economies of scale displaced craft production as the
dominant business model. However, there are still people who
work in the craft mode.

Dashboard

A graphical display of measures important to the success of a
system used to track progress over time.

Deductive Learning

A theory is tested with the aid of a prediction. Observations are
made and any gaps from the prediction based on the theory are
noted and studied. See *Inductive Learning.* Both deductive and
inductive learning are built into the use of the PDSA cycle.

W. Edwards Deming/Dr. Deming

Deming (1900–1993), U.S. statistician and management innovator, was a thought leader of the modern quality movement. After WWII his extensive lectures to Japanese government and industry leaders played a role in helping the Japanese to become a world-class producer of quality products and services. Since 1951 the Deming Prize has been awarded annually to reward Japanese companies for major advances in quality improvement. The awards ceremony is broadcast every year in Japan on national television. In recent years companies outside of Japan have applied for the Deming Prize.

Descriptive Theory

Descriptive theories explain our observations and allow us to hypothesize some correlation; however our theory is weaker at this stage of evolution. Additional testing in our actual circumstances must be done to move the theory into the normative stage.

Detailed Complexity

Immediate cause and effect is understood; take action *x* and *y* happens. See *Dynamic Complexity*.

DRG

Diagnosis-related group (DRG) is a system to classify hospital cases into one of originally 467 groups. The 467th group was the "other" category of cases not lending themselves to be grouped.

Drives

The largely unconscious motivations that are expressed in values and needs that motivate people at work.

Driver Diagram

An approach to describing our theories of improvement. In an improvement project, a driver diagram is a tool to help organize our theories and ideas in an improvement effort as we answer, "What change can we make that will result in improvement?"

The initial driver diagram for an improvement project might lay out the descriptive theory of improved outcomes that can then be tested and enhanced to develop a predictive (normative) theory. The driver diagram should be updated throughout an improvement effort and used to track progress in theory building.

Driver Processes

Those processes that drive the mainstay of the organization. These processes are usually associated with the needs the organization intends to fulfill and usually have a direct impact on the customers of the organization.

Dynamic Complexity

Situations where cause and effect are subtle, and where the effects of interventions over time are not clear. When the same action has dramatically different effects in the short run and the long run, there is dynamic complexity. When an action has one set of consequences locally and a different set of consequences in another part of the system, there is dynamic complexity. When obvious interventions produce nonobvious consequences, there is dynamic complexity.

EBM

Evidence-based medicine, or evidence-based practice (EBP), employs techniques from science, engineering, and statistics to improve diagnosis and clinical treatments.

EHR

Electronic health record.

ESRD

End state renal disease.

Extrinsic Motivation

The satisfaction lies outside the work activity itself and the motivation comes from means other than the work itself.

Extraversion

The tendency within a personality manifested in outgoing, talkative, energetic behavior; versus introversion.

Five Rs

Reasons, **R**esponsibilities, **R**elationships, **R**ewards, and **R**ecognition are designed so that people in an organization are motivated to implement the vision of the organization.

Flow Diagram

A graphic representation of a series of activities that define a process. The diagram shows the stages of a process as inputs are transformed into outcomes.

Foresight

Perception of the significance of events by the leader before they have occurred based on the leader's subject matter expertise, experience, research, scanning, and ability to sense dynamic trends.

Four Ps

Purpose, **P**ractical values, **P**rocesses, and **P**eople interact in an organizational system to describe and achieve the vision.

Fundamental Change

Fundamental changes include the following (also see *Reactive Change*):

- Design or redesign of some aspect of the system
- Necessary for improvement beyond problems
- Fundamentally alters the system and what people do
- Affects several measures in a positive direction; increasing quality while also reducing costs
- Long-term impact

Gap Survey

This survey, originally designed by Michael Maccoby, is used to stimulate engagement, dialogue, and responsibility for improvement. Respondents score each survey item on both its Importance to them and how well the item is currently being practiced. The mean score for each item's How Well Being Practiced is subtracted from the mean for Importance. The difference is the Gap for the item. The Gaps indicate how far an organization is from its ideals in the view of the survey participants.

Hawthorne Effect

The Hawthorne Works of Western Electric was the site of an industrial design experiment in the 1930s. The results are often mistakenly interpreted to mean that any new workplace experiment will result in short-lived productivity gains that last only until the observers leave and the novelty wears off.

Hierarchy of Needs

Abraham Maslow's theory that human need can be described in five levels with each level having to be satisfied before a supposed higher level can be reached and satisfied: (1) physiological needs; (2) safety needs; (3) love and belonging; (4) esteem; and (5) self-actualization.

Idealized Future

The vision of an organization defined operationally in terms of the Four Ps: purpose, practical values, people, and processes.

Identity

The self-definition we choose. Our identity may include physical characteristics and the roles and groups we identify with. Our identity also integrates and gives meaning to our value-drives.

Improvement (see also *Fundamental Change*)

(1) Alters how work or activity is done or the makeup of a product; (2) produces visible, positive differences in results relative to historical norms; and (3) has a lasting impact.

Inductive Learning

The theory of prediction based on observations; for example, predicting the next event based upon observations. The danger of induction: All swans observed are white; therefore all swans are white.

Innovation

Making a change that results in something new and sustainable. The application of knowledge to produce new knowledge; innovation is an important part of improvement through the design of new products and processes.

Interactive Social Character

The social character of people whose attitudes and values motivate them to adapt to a knowledge-service organization. They tend to be other-directed, experimental, innovative, marketing, and they identify with peers and siblings more than with parental authorities; versus the bureaucratic social character.

Interdependence

The mutual dependence and interaction among the elements, people, and processes of a system. Interdependence means that components of a system do not work independently.

Intrinsic Motivation

Wanting to do an activity for the challenge, pleasure, or satisfaction of doing it. The activity engages individuals' values and skills.

Introversion

The tendencies in the personality manifested in more reserved, quiet, and shy behavior; versus extraversion.

Leader

A leader is a person others follow. A leader can be followed out of fear, because the follower is seduced, or persuaded, or because the follower wants to collaborate with the leader to achieve a shared objective.

Leadership Philosophy

The leadership philosophy includes four elements, based on the answers to these questions:

1. What is the purpose of this organization?
2. What ethical and moral reasoning determines the key decisions we make?
3. What practical values do we need to practice to achieve the purpose?
4. How do we define goals and results so they are consistent with our purpose and values?

Leading Indicators

Leading indicators are measures that help to predict outcome measures that are only available periodically. They predict what is likely to happen in the future.

Lean

A production process and redesign discipline that aims to eliminate the expenditure of resources for anything that does not add value for the end customer. Lean aims to drive out waste from the system. The purpose of lean is to create or preserve value with less work and cost. Lean has been popularized based on the work described in the Toyota Production System (TPS). TPS is renowned for its focus on reduction of the original Toyota seven wastes: transportation, inventory, motion, waiting, overprocessing, overproduction, and defects.

Learning Organization

Some defining attributes:

- Developed as a social system where all the parts interact to achieve the purpose of serving patients; designing and redesigning the system of delivering care decreases per capita cost while maintaining or improving patient outcomes.

- Learning from practice is widely shared and used for innovation and improvement: partners with suppliers, client organizations, and community organizations; providers collaborate across disciplines, with patients and their families.
- Learning is used to inform the community, aid in the prevention of illness, and improve population health.

Leverage

Used to identify where actions and fundamental changes can take place in a system which can lead to a large sustainable impact on system measures and outcomes.

LOS

Length of stay is a term used to measure the duration of hospitalization for patients. Inpatient days are calculated by subtracting day of admission from day of discharge. A popular statistic associated with length of stay is the average length of stay (ALOS), calculated by dividing the sum of inpatient days by the number of patient admissions with the same DRG classification.

Mainstay Process

Those processes that directly relate to the mission of the organization and add value to the external customers of the organization.

Manufacturing Mode of Production

The manufacturing mode of production describes a way of organizing work and relationships based on producing standardized and replaceable product parts, fragmentation of work into simplified tasks, workers hired for the repetition of these tasks, and the bureaucratization of the functions that support the assembly process. Beginning with time and motion studies the science of reducing labor and material use led to significant efficiencies of production. The manufacturing mode eventually spread to service and government work.

Mistake 1—Type 1 Error

A mistake made in an attempt to improve results in which an outcome is reacted to as if it came from a special cause, when actually it came from common causes of variation.

Mistake 2—Type 2 Error

A mistake made in an attempt to improve results in which an outcome is treated as if it came from common causes of variation, when actually it came from a special cause.

Mode of Production

The organization of work based on a particular system of the tools, values, knowledge, relationships, and attitudes that are essential to produce particular products.

Model for Improvement

The Model for Improvement contains two basic components:

1. Three questions needed to guide any improvement or change effort
2. The Plan-Do-Study-Act (PDSA) cycle

The Model is a flexible framework for focused questions and, if appropriate, the use of application-specific tools and methodology. The three questions are

1. What are we trying to accomplish?
2. How will we know that a change is an improvement?
3. What change can we make that will result in improvement?

Moral Reasoning

Laurence Kohlberg described three levels of moral reasoning:

1. The lowest level defines the good as individual well-being, avoiding punishment or gaining rewards.
2. The next level defines the good in terms of what a person considers good for family or organization as well as for him- or herself, without concern for the effect of his or her actions on others.

3. A broader definition of the common good is what benefits, or at least doesn't harm, all those who may be affected by one's actions: employees, customers, owners, communities, unborn generations, and the natural environment.

Motivation

What makes a person act. Motivation can be caused by intrinsic drives and values or extrinsic incentives.

Motivational Type

The personality types that can be viewed as motivational systems, representing patterns of value-drives. In each type, one or more value-drives are dominant and determine the strongest motivational values of that type. Described by Freud, Fromm, Maccoby, and Porter.

Network Leader

A network leader facilitates collaboration across the organization, disciplines, processes, and roles. Network leaders are followed because of their ability to bring people together to accomplish shared tasks, irrespective of where they are in the organization.

Normative Theory

Normative theories predict the results we can expect from changing the way things are done. When the predictions are correct, our theory is confirmed. If the observed results prove the prediction incorrect, we want to understand why, so that the categorization can be updated, made more precise, or the theory abandoned. Good theory building demands that we test to disconfirm theories rather than to test merely to confirm by determining under what circumstances our theory proves incorrect.

OCHIN

Our Community Healthcare Information Network is a collaborative provider for health records technology, research, and innovative care solutions in thirteen states.

Operational Definition

Operational definitions are necessary to create shared meaning. An operational definition should include (1) a method of measurement or test; (2) a set of criteria for judgment.

Operational Leader

An operational leader is a person who leads the design and management of processes. Ideally, operational leaders work interactively with strategic and network leaders to achieve the organization's purpose.

Partnering

The process that involves a person or organization associated with others in a relationship focused on achieving a common purpose. A partner participates in a relationship where each member has equal status while working together for the shared purpose. The book identifies a continuum of levels of partnering relationships.

PDSA Cycle

PDSA (Plan-Do-Study-Act) is a methodology for learning from data and the experience of developing, testing, and implementing changes. It is a component of the Model for Improvement.

Personality

A systems concept that describes the structure of a person's intellect, drives, and values. Personality, arising in childhood, is relatively permanent over the person's life. However, an individual can develop his or her personality to become more productive. Personality explains our unconscious and conscious motivations, satisfactions, relationships, and ways of working. For example, the personality types visionary, caring, exacting, and adapting describe different patterns of value-drives.

Personality Intelligence

Understanding of the personalities of oneself and others, including values that drive behavior at work. Understanding the people you lead means that you are aware of their identities, strengths, motivations, and emotions. This requires learning concepts that sensitize you to patterns of behavior and developing your heart as well as your intellect.

Practical Values

The values required to achieve a leader's or an organization's purpose. Practical values are sometimes called guiding principles, targeted behaviors, shared values, operational values.

Process

A set of causes and conditions that repeatedly come together in a sequential series of steps to transform inputs into outcomes.

Process Improvement

The continuous study of the cause-and-effect mechanisms in a process in order to reduce variation, remove complexity, optimize important quality characteristics, and thereby improve customer satisfaction.

Profound Knowledge

A concept developed by W. Edwards Deming to understand and optimize organizations. The system of profound knowledge has four parts: appreciation of a system, understanding variation, theory of knowledge, and psychology.

Project Charter Approval Form

This form is designed to communicate the purpose of a team or individual involved in an improvement effort and spells out what is trying to be accomplished, who has responsibilities to do each part of the process, and how results will be measured. This form facilitates answering the first two questions in the Model for Improvement: (1) What are we trying to accomplish? (2) How will we know that a change is an improvement?

Project Charter

The project charter helps teams and individuals manage their efforts and reduce unwanted variations from the original aim as well as know when they have completed their project. The charter is usually framed around the three questions related to the Model for Improvement.

Purpose

Purpose describes why the organization exists and how the organization meets its obligations to customers. A powerful statement of purpose will be meaningful to all stakeholders. Many organizations use *mission* to describe the organization's purpose.

Quality

The concept of the ongoing match of products and services to a need, with the customer defining the characteristics for matching. Deming defined quality as "whatever the customer says it is."

Qulturum

An organization in Jönköping, Sweden, that drives learning and change with a strategic purpose and develops individuals to apply learning and achieve improved results for the system. It is a learning center and meeting point where employees use action-based training in order to improve their respective skills. The name itself is defined as qultur—culture—soil for change:

Q—quality
U—utveckling, improvement
L—leadership
T
U
R
UM—ends words in Latin that describes people and gatherings, such as forum, centrum, agorum

Reactive Change

Reactive changes can be characterized by the following attributes:

- Solve problems or react
- Return the system to prior condition

- Tradeoff among measures; increasing quality while increasing costs
- Short-term impact

Rules for Special Causes

1. A single point outside the control limits. 2. A run of eight or more points in a row above (or below) the centerline. 3. Six consecutive points increasing (trend up) or decreasing (trend down). 4. Two out of three consecutive points near (outer one-third) a control limit. 5. Fifteen consecutive points close (inner one-third of the chart) to the centerline. See Figure 7.2 for a graphic of each special cause type.

Run Chart

A graphical record of a quality characteristic measured over time. That is, a measure of quality from a work process plotted on a graph so its variation can be studied and improvements made in the process.

Seven Value-Drives

There are seven types of innate drives that through socialization become our emotionally charged needs and values, which Maccoby has called value-drives: survival, relatedness, mastery, information, play, dignity, meaning.

Shared Identity

An effective leader not only recognizes the importance of creating a shared identity that communicates a philosophy with a purpose that inspires people, but that leader also describes and practices the values essential to achieve that purpose. These values, such as quality care, efficiency, and collaboration, will connect with the values of people in the organization.

Walter Shewhart

An American physicist, engineer, and statistician (1891–1967) considered the father of statistical quality (or process) control. Shewhart developed the control chart technique which is often called the "Shewhart Chart."

Single- and Double-Loop Learning

Single-loop learning occurs when the results of our practice don't fit the theory and we interpret this as a need to change or fine tune our practice. An example would be a physician making a diagnosis, and finding that the indicated treatment did not produce the expected result. The physician does not question the theory in single-loop learning, but assumes that he or she didn't perform the treatment correctly. With double-loop learning, the physician questions the diagnosis and treatment and is open to new information that can lead to changing the underlying theory and assumptions. The concept was developed by Chris Argyris.

Social Character

That part of a person's personality shared with others raised to adapt to a particular culture and mode of production. The social character adapts people to survive economically and emotionally in that culture. Fromm's concept of social character expanded Freud's largely intrapsychic model of personality, and Maccoby applied it to the shift from the craft and bureaucratic to the interactive social character now occurring in society and organizations.

Special Cause

Those causes *not* part of the process (or system) all the time or that do not affect everyone, but arise because of specific circumstances. The elimination of special causes allows a system to become a predictable and stable system.

Sponsor Report

A one-page report used by the team or individual making an improvement to communicate to the sponsor. The sponsor of the improvement project is kept in the communication loop by receiving regular updates on the sponsor report.

Stable

A system is stable when it has only common causes affecting the outcomes, or it is in a state of statistical control. A stable process implies only that the variation is predictable from the data displayed on a control chart.

Stakeholder

A person or group that has a stake in an organization. Stakeholders include the community, employees, professional associations, unions, boards, and governments, among others.

SPC (Statistical Process Control)

Usually philosophy and a set of methods for improvement with its foundation in the theory of variation. SPC incorporates the concepts of an analytic study, process thinking, prevention, stratification, stability, capability, and prediction. Tools such as run charts, control charts, flow diagrams, histograms, Pareto charts, scatterplots, and cause-and-effect diagrams are typically associated with SPC. Kaoru Ishikawa, at the time an associate professor at the University of Tokyo, called these the Seven Basic Tools of Quality Control.

Strategic Intelligence

The qualities that equip a leader of change. It is a conceptual system, described by Michael Maccoby, consisting of foresight, visioning (with systems thinking and idealized design), partnering, and motivating. Each of these elements interacts with the others. Like any type of intelligence there is a genetic basis or inherent talent at birth. No matter the extent of this inherent gift, it can be developed to some extent through learning and practice. A leader's effectiveness in applying strategic intelligence depends on his or her leadership philosophy, personality intelligence, and analytical, creative, and practical intelligences. Strategic intelligence is strengthened by a leadership philosophy and profound knowledge.

Strategic Leader

A leader who defines purpose and vision, aligning people, processes, and practical values so they support and further the organization's purpose. Although effective strategic leaders may not have all the qualities of strategic intelligence, they partner with others so that these qualities exist among members of their leadership team. A strategic leader can be at any level of an organization. Ideally, the top executives are strategic leaders.

Support Process

Those processes that are necessary to support the mainstay and driver processes in the organization viewed as a system. Examples typically include accounting processes, maintenance, hiring, traveling, and scheduling.

System

A collection of elements that work interactively to achieve a purpose. There are mechanical systems that can be designed, organic systems that are determined genetically and social systems that must be designed and led. Definition of a social system with the Four Ps as a foundation: a collection of interdependent *processes* and other elements with *people* working interactively guided by *practical values* to accomplish the *purpose* of the system.

Systems Map

The graphic depiction of the levels of the organization that shows the linkage of processes for the whole organization. These maps typically include three types of processes: mainstay (delivery system to the customer), support, and driver processes.

Systems Thinking

The ability to understand the dynamics between the parts of a system and aligning them so that they interact to achieve the system's purpose; using systems thinking principles, such as system boundaries, bottlenecks, constraints, leverage, and appreciating that all work is a process.

Tertiary Care

Highly specialized medical care, usually over an extended period of time, that involves advanced and complex procedures and treatments performed by medical specialists. Major hospitals that provide tertiary care usually have a full complement of services including pediatrics; obstetrics; neurology; general medicine; gynecology; various branches of surgery, including trauma surgery; and psychiatry.

Theory Building

Theories are developed as we experience and observe events. Theory building is the process of making theories more accurate and effective. The process of theory building takes place in two stages: descriptive theory and normative theory. In the first stage of theory building, we describe phenomena and suggest associations. At some point in the theory building process, the statements of theory switch from association (descriptive) to causation (normative).

Transparency

Sharing information about costs, revenues, and investments with stakeholders to achieve engagement, trust, and contribute to solutions. With financial transparency, everyone can be assured that resources are used productively.

Triple Aim

The three aims of health care arose from the work of the Institute for Healthcare Improvement (IHI) and the leadership of Don Berwick. IHI states: "Improving the U.S. health care system requires simultaneous pursuit of three aims: improving the experience of care, improving the health of populations, and reducing per capita costs of health care. Preconditions for this include the enrollment of an identified population, a commitment to universality for its members, and the existence of an organization (an "integrator") that accepts responsibility for all three aims for that population."[2]

Unstable

An unstable system does not necessarily mean one with large variation. Unstable means that the magnitude of the variation from one time period to the next is unpredictable; it is dominated by special cause variation.

Values

Those largely conscious motivations that we make part of our identity and seek to achieve through our philosophy of life, such as security, love, innovation, excellence.

Visioning

Designing the idealized future of the organization as a learning organization that can innovate and take account of the trends seen by foresight that indicate threats or opportunities for the organization. This book describes the visioning process of defining and implementing a strategic vision as a systemic blueprint of an ideal future that would achieve the organization's purpose more effectively and efficiently.

ENDNOTES

1. Charles Van Doren and Mortimer J. Adler, *How to Read a Book* (New York: Touchstone), Kindle edition, 96–97.
2. Donald M. Berwick, Thomas W. Nolan, and John Whittington, "The Triple Aim: Care, Health, and Cost," *Health Affairs* 27, no. 3 (2008): 759–769. Also available from http://content.healthaffairs.org/content/27/3/759.full.pdf.html

Index

Page numbers in italics refer to figures, tables, and exhibits.